NURSING CARE PLANS

SERIES EDITORS

Kathleen M Berry SRN SCM RNT AcDipEd
Will Bridge BSc PhD
Jill Macleod Clark BSc SRN

In the same series

Research for Nursing — A Guide for the Enquiring Nurse
Teaching Patient Care — A Handbook for the Practising Nurse
Communication in Nursing Care

EDUCATION FOR CARE

Nursing Care Plans
The Nursing Process at Work

JENNIFER M HUNT MPhil BA SRN
Director of Nursing Research,
The Royal Marsden Hospital, London

DIANE J MARKS-MARAN BSc SRN Dip N(Lond)
Ward Sister,
The Royal Marsden Hospital, London

Foreword by
BARONESS McFARLANE OF LLANDAFF
FRCN MA MSc SRN SCM HVTCert
Professor and Head of Department of Nursing
University of Manchester

An HM + M Nursing Publication

JOHN WILEY & SONS

Chichester · New York · Brisbane · Toronto · Singapore

HM + M is an imprint of JOHN WILEY & SONS LTD

ISBN 0 471 25778 8

Typeset by Inforum Ltd., Portsmouth
Printed in Great Britain by Mackays of Chatham Ltd, Lordswood,
Chatham, Kent

Contents

Foreword

Many nurses will welcome this book. Not only has there been a lack of English literature about the nursing process at work but English nurses have wanted very practical guidance on how to set about using the nursing process, how it will affect their work and above all, what kind of records they will need to develop.

The authors have had a very practical involvement in all this. That is why they can speak with authority on the design and use of nursing history forms and every other stage of the process.

I am delighted with this book because it not only gives us some very practical tools which have been tested, but it gives us the honour of being treated as professional people in our own right. We are not just left with the authors' work as the definitive statement about the nursing process – we are introduced to some theoretical considerations which are the basis of the use of the nursing process and given a liberal list of further reading. The nurse who is striving towards excellence in nursing care will, I am sure, not just want to rake over the work here published, but will want to take it further and build on what has already been developed.

McFarlane of Llandaff
April 1980

Preface

This book is about the nursing process at work, through the development and use of *Nursing Care Plans*. We call this implementation of the nursing process *care planning*. Our aim is to provide a guide to this approach which is relevant to both the hospital and community settings in the United Kingdom and which also enables nurses to plan care around the individual needs of each patient. We hope that trained staff and learners who are interested in and wish to initiate and practise care planning will find it useful and that they will put what they learn into practice for the benefit of the patient.

During the last decade nurses have become increasingly aware of the need for a more systematic approach to nursing care. This awareness results from a number of factors which include a desire to identify and establish 'nursing' as a profession with its own body of knowledge; concern about standards of care; and the need to keep nursing records which will provide an accurate detailed account of the patient's stay in hospital. At the same time nurses do not want to lose their caring rôle, for this rôle is central to nursing. Care planning provides the basis for a systematic approach to nursing care and emphasises the uniquely caring aspects of nursing.

A great deal has been written recently about the nursing process, but it is not always obvious how nurses should use it. We have put it to work in care planning since it provides a framework within which all nursing can take place.

The nursing process is usually divided into four stages: assessment; planning; implementation and evaluation. The importance of accurate written records is emphasised for each of these stages to provide the information needed to determine the effectiveness of the care provided. Nursing care planning uses these same four stages.

The nursing process and care planning should, and can, complement each other. If nursing is to develop and grow it is vital that theory should be translated into practice and that practice should be based on theory. However, definitions alone cannot provide nurses with practical guidelines on how the nursing process can be implemented. This lack of guidance has proved a major drawback to its clinical use in the United Kingdom and this book attempts to redress the balance by drawing together the concepts relating to the nursing process and demonstrating how these concepts can be used effectively in the clinical setting.

In this book we explain our views on the nursing process and care planning on the basis of our experience at The London Hospital and the Royal Marsden Hospital. Our approach will not suit everyone. We do not claim that it is the only way of implementing care planning. However, we do believe that it is a good approach which can be adapted for use in both hospital and community. Above all it provides nurses with an exciting and challenging opportunity to assess the effectiveness of the care that they give to their patients and to improve this care when necessary.

We believe that the opportunity to implement the nursing process and introduce care planning must not be missed. Both have been written about and talked about a great deal in recent years. It is now time to act. All kinds of discussions are taking place as nurses look for ways in which they can improve the care they give to patients. Care planning is one of these ways and one in which every nurse can and should become involved.

Jennifer M Hunt
Diane Marks-Maran
London, January 1980

Acknowledgements

We would like to thank all those who have helped us to write this book. In particular we would like to thank Miss M Day and the other members of the Nursing Research Steering Committee for their encouragement and support of the research project which started us off, the N E Thames Regional Health Authority for providing the grant which made it possible, the nurses at The London Hospital and the Royal Marsden Hospital who were willing to try using the Nursing Care Plans, and the Editor of the *Nursing Times* for permission to use material first published in that journal. Our especial thanks must go to all those friends who have helped by listening, discussing and arguing.

Finally, we would like to express our gratitude for the help we received from members of the Editorial Board and from the secretaries who typed and re-typed the manuscript.

Jennifer M Hunt
Diane Marks-Maran
January 1980

What are Nursing Care Plans?

Nursing Care Plans are written for individual patients and are a practical way of putting the nursing process to work. They are not the same thing as the nursing process, although there is a definite relationship between the activity of producing Nursing Care Plans and the philosophy of the nursing process. Producing a Nursing Care Plan involves assessing the patient's needs and planning appropriate care. The nursing care can then be given, or modified and adapted as necessary, using the written record called the Nursing Care Plan; furthermore, care given can subsequently be evaluated. A Nursing Care Plan is, therefore, a practical tool which helps nurses to give individualised care to patients.

A Nursing Care Plan has four purposes. It provides an assessment of the patient's needs; details of the planned care; a description of how this was implemented, and an evaluation of the outcomes for the patient. These steps correspond to the four stages of the nursing process. Learning about Nursing Care Plans, and gaining practice in their use, should help nurses towards a clearer understanding of the principles of the nursing process.

It is important that readers should understand the terminology which has been used throughout the book, to avoid the danger of confusion. When we talk about *Nursing Care Plans,* (ie. capital initial letters and preceded by Nursing) we mean all the paperwork which is needed to put the nursing process to work, including the patient's history, his progress notes, and the planned programme of patient care itself.

However, when we speak of the whole process of decision-making and recording which is necessary in order to produce a Nursing Care Plan, we have termed this activity *care planning* (ie. without 'nursing' and without capital initials). On occasion, particularly in Chapters 3 and 5, we will need to refer to that part of the whole Nursing Care Plan which contains just the written list of the patient's problems, and corresponding actions and goals. We have called this document the *Care Plan,* but wherever we have used this phrase we have differentiated it from the whole Nursing Care Plan.

Introduction

The purpose of this book is to provide a basic guide to care planning and to give practical help in making the nursing process a reality at ward level. The book is divided into three sections, of which the first provides an introduction to Nursing Care Plans and gives a background to using them and the nursing process generally. In this section, we also discuss different types of ward management and organising patient care; task allocation, team nursing and patient allocation. There is also a chapter describing our own experiences at The London Hospital and how we began to use Nursing Care Plans.

The second section takes the four stages of the nursing process (assessment, planning, implementation and evaluation) and discusses how each stage can be fitted into the Nursing Care Plan. The third section contains a list of hints and ideas which we offer to help nurses when beginning to use Nursing Care Plans, and we end our book with a reading guide for nurses who would like to extend their knowledge of care planning; a detailed bibliography is also included in this section.

Throughout the book we try to emphasise the practical aspects of care planning, including our successes as well as the mistakes we made. We hope you will find using Nursing Care Plans and the nursing process exciting, as well as practically valuable, in terms of giving good patient care.

Section I

An Introduction to Nursing Care Plans

In this first section we take an overall look at care planning, placing it within the theoretical framework of the nursing process. We then turn to the practical problem of how to integrate care planning into the ward setting by discussing its relationship to three methods of organising care; task allocation, team nursing, and patient allocation. This discussion makes clear our belief that care planning and patient allocation cannot be separated. Finally, we describe our experiences in trying care planning at The London Hospital in order to illustrate how theory can be put into practice. We have tried to illuminate not just the problems but also the benefits we gained from our work in this field.

Chapter 1

Words and Meanings

Here we discuss the development of nursing care planning and its relationship to the nursing process, the stages of care planning, and the format and design of Nursing Care Plans. Based on our experience we show how the ideas and concepts of care planning can be applied to, and successfully used in the ward.

> "The unique function of the professional nurse may be conceived to be (1) the identification of the *nursing* problem and (2) the deciding upon of a course of nursing actions to be followed for the solution of the problem in the light of immediate and long-term objectives of nursing." MCMANUS (1950).

> "Patient care planning is the systematic assessment and identification of problems, the setting of objectives and the establishment of methods and strategies for accomplishing them." MAYERS (1972).

Looking at the above quotations, it would seem that care planning is not new. Its use and usefulness have in fact come about over a long period of time. At first, it was used mainly as an educational tool by teaching staff but recent developments have concentrated on its use on the wards. Only when care planning is used by all nurses working both in hospital and the community will its benefits be fully realised and appreciated.

It is very important first of all to define the terms we will be using:

> *Care planning*   A systematic approach to planning patient care which enables the nurse to obtain all the information she requires to provide effective nursing care which will meet the individual needs of the patient.

> *Nursing Care Plans*   The visible and written record of the

implementation of care planning. They document the use of this approach. A Nursing Care Plan has 3 components: nursing history, Care Plan and progress record.

The nursing process   The theoretical framework for the development of care planning.

Both care planning and the nursing process are usually divided into four steps: assessment, planning, implementation and evaluation. It is very important not to confuse Step 2 of the nursing process, planning (Chapter 5), with the Nursing Care Plans themselves.

Why we need nursing care planning

Nursing in the United Kingdom has traditionally revolved around a task allocation approach to clinical care, ie. nursing care has been described as 'the work' and lists of jobs to be done were written. Very few nursing actions have been laid open to a close look at what is being done and why it is being done; there have been few, if any, scientific principles behind nursing care. Care planning uses a problem-solving approach. This emphasis on problem solving should encourage nurses to develop a much more objective and logical approach to their work.

While the development of the medical profession has been built upon research, with changes and improvements being made as new ideas and knowledge arise, this is not so in nursing. Relatively little nursing research has been carried out in the UK, but even where studies have been undertaken the information obtained is seldom put to use in the clinical setting. This may be due to the fact that nurses are unaware that such information is available. Also, nursing care is seldom evaluated and continues to centre on nursing activities developed from medical diagnoses, rather than on the individual nursing needs of the patient or on research information. Phrases commonly heard on wards such as "the appendicectomy in Bed 10" or "all our herniorrhaphies have x, y and z done to them" or "use lotion X because Sister likes it" bear witness to this fact.

One of the factors which allow medical staff to evaluate the treatment of their patients' condition is the medical record, which forms a permanent and continuous picture of the patient's medical treatment. This is particularly true when Problem-Oriented Medical Records (POMR) are used. Nothing is erased in the medical record as the treatment changes, and general phrases, so common in the nurses' Kardex record system, do not exist. Changes in the patient's condition are noted and new plans of treatment are written and subsequently evaluated. Although nurses have some record in the Kardex of their care of the patient, these recordings are frequently little more than "slept well"; "specimen of urine N.A.D; good day; up and about". These phrases give no real indication of the patient's progress, nor of the care that he has been given or how effective is the care.

Nursing care planning and the nursing process Care planning has recently become closely associated with, and an integral part of, what is called the nursing process. Many nurses, however, dislike this term because it is seen as being too high-powered or meaningless, and are using other though similar terms to describe planning care, for example, 'individualised care planning' or 'total patient care'. Traditionally, nursing has had a practical emphasis. Practical rather than theoretical ability has been stressed , and in fact, nurses who do take a more questioning, thinking approach are often discouraged from doing so. The development of a theory of nursing which will involve both thinking and questioning is, however, very important if nursing is to take its rightful place alongside medicine as a profession which provides for the needs of patients. The nursing process emphasises the importance of practical nursing skills — it certainly does not deny these as some nurses believe, but also makes nurses think more about what they are doing, why they are doing it and whether or not it is working.

Nursing care theory It is not the intention of this book to be a theoretical text, although the theory underlying the nursing process and the planning of individualised care is dealt with briefly in Chapter 8. For those who wish to pursue a more theoretical approach or obtain knowledge of the subject in depth a comprehensive bibliography has been included in Section IV.

The model (Fig. 1) devised by Hunt (1975) shows that ideally there should be complete similarity between:

> the nursing care which has been prescribed
> that which has been given, and
> that which the patient needs.

A problem-orientated approach to planning and implementing

nursing care works towards achieving this similarity by identifying the patient's individual needs and then planning the nursing action required.

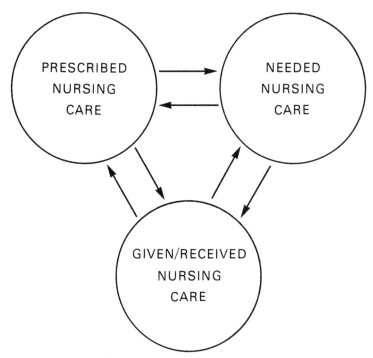

Fig. 1   Nursing care: a theoretical model

The importance of written records

In order to be effective, the planning of care must be expressed in a permanent form. This is achieved through the development of a written Nursing Care Plan which is a continuous, comprehensive record of the nursing care a patient should receive and the care he has received. (A Nursing Care Plan which is erased as changes occur is not a permanent record.) A Nursing Care Plan should include the following components:

Information about the patient   Nursing History
(Fig. 2)

NURSING HISTORY

Record Number _____	Consultant _____
PATIENT LABEL	House Officer _____
Name _____	Diagnosis _____
Address _____	_____
_____	_____
_____	_____
Date of Birth _____ Age _____	Operations on present admission
Date of Admission _____ Time _____	_____
Type: Emergency Planned	_____
Transfer from _____	_____
Marital status _____ Religion _____	_____
Next of Kin (Name) _____	Past medical history/operations ___
Relationship to Patient _____	_____
Address _____	_____
_____	_____
_____	_____
Tel. No(s) _____	_____
_____	_____
_____	Allergies _____
Speech difficulty/language barrier	_____
	History of present complaint _____
Care at home: Details/Names	_____
Community Nurse _____	_____
Social Worker _____	_____
Social Services _____	Other current health problems ____
(Please state _____	_____
specific service) _____	What *patient* says is the reason f
G.P. (Name) _____	_____
_____	_____
_____	_____
_____	_____

Fig. 2   The nursing history (sheet 1)

	NURSING REMINDERS _____
	_____
	_____
	_____
	_____
	SOCIAL HISTORY Occupation_____
date performed	Children_____
	Other dependants_____
	HOUSING (House, flat – which floor, stairs,
	lives alone, shares, bathroom/toilet)_____
	_____
	_____
	_____
	_____
	_____
	Other problems at home?_____
	Visiting problems? Yes No
	If Yes, describe:_____
	DISCHARGE PLANNING (Please tick those required and add the date when they are ordered or done

	Needed	Date ordered
Social Services – specify	_____	_____
	_____	_____
	_____	_____
Community Nurse	_____	_____
TTA's and Teaching	_____	_____
Out-patients' appt.	_____	_____
Transport	_____	_____
Relatives informed	_____	_____
Other	_____	_____

admission_____

DAILY LIVING		HEARING	Right:	Good
DIET			Left:	Good
Special_____ _____		Hearing Aid?	Yes	No
Food or drink dislikes:_____		Remarks_____		
_____		**VISION**	Right:	Good
Appetite: Good Poor			Left:	Good
Remarks_____			Glasses	
_____		Remarks_____		
SLEEP How many hours usually?_____		**PROSTHESIS/APPLIANCE/AIDS**		
Sedation_____		Type(s)_____		
Other comments_____		_____		
ELIMINATION				
BOWELS: Any problems: Yes No		Any help needed? Yes		
If Yes, describe_____		**MOBILITY** Fully mobile?		
_____		If no – needs help with:		
How often are bowels opened?_____		Walking Standing		
_____		Washing Bathing		
Any medication?_____		In/Out of bed In/Out of chair		
URINARY: No problems Incontinence		_____		
Nocturia Dysuria		_____		
Frequency Urgency		_____		
Remarks_____		**ORAL**		
_____		Any problems with mouth or teeth?		
FEMALE PATIENTS – MENSTRUATION		If Yes, describe_____		
Regular Irregular		Wears dentures? Yes N		
Amenorrhoea Dysmenorrhoea		_____		
Post-Menopausal Taking the Pill		Any problems with dentures?_____		
Next period due_____		_____		
Will need: ST's Tampons		_____		
Remarks_____		Any crowns?_____		
Information obtained: From_____ By _____				

Fig. 2   The nursing history (sheet 2)

Poor	Deaf	
Poor	Deaf	
Poor	Blind	
Poor	Blind	
Contact Lenses		
No		
Yes	No	
Dressing		
Feeding		
Other ___		
Yes	No	
Upper	Lower	

NURSES OBSERVATIONS

ATTITUDE

Anxious   Withdrawn   Distressed

Remarks – (If particular problem please try and state reason e.g.

anxious about operation/or being in hospital etc. ___

___

___

___

___

GENERAL APPEARANCE

Normal   Obese

Dehydrated   Thin

Acutely ill   Emaciated

Remarks___

___

___

SKIN

Satisfactory   Broken areas

Dehydrated   Rash

Oedematous   Jaundiced

Describe___

___

LEVEL OF CONCIOUSNESS

Orientated   Semi-conscious

Confused   Unconscious

Remarks___

___

___

Level of training/position ___

Date   Time

CARE PLAN			

DISCHARGE GOALS

DISCHARGE PLANNING

Tick those needed   Dat

Social services

Community nursing

TTA's and teaching

Out-patients' appt.

Transport

Other _____

DATE	NO	PATIENT'S NURSING NEEDS/PROBLEMS AND CAUSES OF PROBLEMS (N B Physiological, Psychological, Social and Family problems)	

Fig. 3   The Care Plan

rdered

OUTCOMES/RESULTS OF NURSING CARE

GOALS	NURSING INSTRUCTIONS	REVIEW ON/BY	DATE RESOLVED

DATE	SHIFT	PROGRESS NOTES

WARD: BED NO:

Fig. 4 The progress record

RESPONSIBLE NURSE (initials)	NURSING CARE TO BE COMPLETED OR CARRIED OUT DURING NEXT SPAN OF DUTY
NAME:	

Identification of the patient's actual
  or likely nursing problems   Care Plan
                                            (Fig 3.)

Patient-centred goals for each problem

Specific nursing instructions to
  achieve these goals

A report on the patient's progress
  in relation to each problem   Progress Record
                                            (Fig. 4)

Evaluation of the nursing action   Care Plan and
                                            Progress Record

A care plan is centred on the patient and is specifically written
for that patient — ideally with his help. The Nursing Care Plan
takes into account the patient's background and environment,
his likes and dislikes, his response to his illness and his ability to
cope both with his illness and with his daily life. A Nursing Care
Plan is so individual that it cannot be used for any patient other
than the one for whom it was written. Each Nursing Care Plan
therefore is unique.

A Nursing Care Plan should be in continuous use, being
updated as often as any changes occur. It should not be something which is written down on the day of admission and then put
aside and left unchanged and unused. Because of this updating
the Nursing Care Plan contains all the most relevant information
about the patient and therefore accurately reflects his condition
at any time. Because a Nursing Care Plan is a written plan, it is
available to all those involved in the care of the patient both as an
aid to making decisions about future care and in assessing the
effect of care already given to that patient. A Nursing Care Plan
then becomes the basis for ward reporting sessions.

What form should Nursing Care Plans take?

The type of format used will vary from one ward or community
setting to another according to the needs of the patients. Nursing
staff have to be educated into thinking about nursing care in a
more professional and individual way. Part of the problem in
introducing Nursing Care Plans is the discomfort felt by nurses
on having to think about the reasons for the care that they are
giving and on having to consider whether it is what the patient
wants or needs at the time. It also means abandoning some old

ideas about ward routine. Such thinking involves change and change is uncomfortable.

The difference between Nursing Care Plans and work sheets   A Nursing Care Plan is different from a pre-printed instruction sheet or card. Pre-printed cards or sheets contain headings of care (Fig. 5) which are ticked or completed in pencil. Updating is carried out as necessary by erasing the old instructions and replacing them with new. Such an instruction sheet does provide an individual record of current nursing orders for each patient and is very useful for that purpose, but it is not a Nursing Care Plan because it is not a permanent and complete record and lists only a series of erased and updated instructions. This means that the evaluation phase of care planning (which we will show to be very important) is impossible. Care can only be evaluated when the instructions are permanent and the patient's progress is recorded day by day.

Getting started

Like most projects which involve trying out something new or different, particularly when the benefits are not immediately apparent, writing a Nursing Care Plan presents the problem of where to begin. "This is just more writing" or "I've been planning care for ages, why should I write it down?" or "I'm too busy nursing patients to write Nursing Care Plans" are all reasons given by nurses for not wanting to start them. These are really just excuses and not valid reasons at all. Anyone can start — all that is really needed is the desire to do so and a willingness to expend some time and effort, especially in the beginning.

Writing a Nursing Care Plan is really a simple procedure once the basic steps are known and understood, especially problem identification and the setting of goals (Fig. 6). It is simple because the steps are logical, building upon one another in an organised way. Many nurses think along the lines of care planning, but usually their approach is neither systematic nor problem-orientated. Producing a Nursing Care Plan involves using these thought processes to identify and plan care, to solve or relieve nursing problems, and then putting their thoughts down on paper for all members of the health care team to see and use. This is particularly important in situations where learners or inexperienced nurses will be responsible for giving much of the care. By

NURSING INSTRUCTION CARD		Complete in PENCIL	Update AT LEAST once each shift
NURSING CARE PROCEDURES		PREPARATION for OPERATION/INVESTIGATION	INVESTIGATIONS/TREATMENTS
Blanket Bath	By nurse		
Bath/Shower	Assisted		
Wash	Supervised	OBSERVATION: specify frequency	MOBILITY/ACTIVITY
Bowl	By patient	T.P.R.	Bed Rest	To lie flat
Pressure area care:		Blood Pressure	Up in chair	May walk
Frequency		Neurological	Allowed up for: (Specify length of time)
Turn pattern		Weight	Morning
Other instructions		Test Urine	Afternoon
			Evening
Oral toilet		DIET	Allowed to walk:
		Type: (Give details)	From/to
Catheter toilet			Supervised/helped by
Dressings		Help needed:	Other exercise
		FLUIDS	SPECIMENS
		Fluid Chart			Urine
		Restrict	Extra	Stool
Intra-venous care		Amount	mls in 24 hrs	Sputum
		'a' - 0800-1600	mls	Other
Other		'b' - 1600-2200	mls	
		'c' - 2200-0800	mls	
		Frequency		
Name		Bed No.	Nurse

Fig. 5   A nursing instruction card (front)

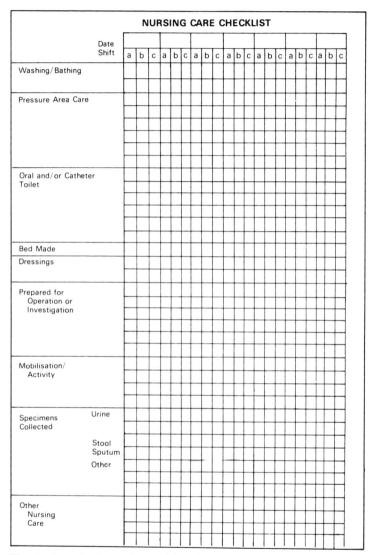

Fig. 5   A nursing instruction card (back)

using this method of documentation they can find out easily what care is prescribed, the reasons for specific nursing action and what that action should achieve as far as the patient is concerned.

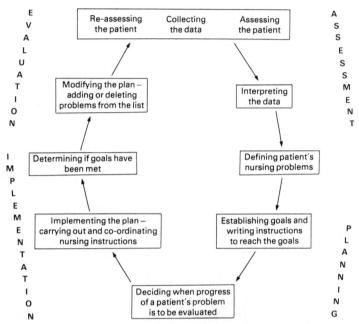

Fig. 6   Development of a problem-orientated Care Plan based on the nursing process

What will Nursing Care Plans achieve?

There is no such thing as a perfect Nursing Care Plan, nor will one 'cure' an incurable problem. Even the best plan cannot ensure that the patient will receive effective care. Good Nursing Care Plans come with knowledge, with practice and with experience. Mistakes or omissions in one Nursing Care Plan should mean that the same mistakes or omissions do not occur the next time round. Success in solving a particular nursing problem should mean that this approach can be used the next time the same problem occurs. This application of information — the avoidance of mistakes, the use of successful methods — cannot be anything but beneficial to the patient because it ensures that he receives the most effective care. The problem-orientated approach challenges many of our accepted practices and procedures, and in its implementation it is bound to challenge more. It is a challenge we should and can meet, and we should enjoy doing so for it will provide us with the means of enabling nurses to achieve their full potential in caring for patients. Such improved care can only raise the standards of the nursing profession.

References

Hunt J. M. (1975) *The Nursing Care Project.* Tower Hamlets Health District. Unpublished report

Mayers M. (1978) *A Systematic Approach to Nursing Care Plans.* New York: Appleton-Century-Crofts

McManus R. (1952) Assumption of functions of nursing. In *Regional Planning for Nursing and Nursing Education.* Report of Conference, Plymouth, New Hampshire, 1950. New York: Columbia University Teachers' College Bureau of Publications

Chapter 2

Ward Organisation and Nursing Care Plans

Care Plans have to fit into the ward organisation, which is by no means uniform. Within a ward there are three ways of organising patient care: task allocation, team nursing and patient allocation. An understanding of the differences between these three methods of allocating nursing duties is necessary before any detailed discussion of care planning can take place.

What is task allocation?

Task allocation is the assignment of individual and not necessarily related jobs or tasks to a particular nurse. For example, Student Nurse Smith takes all the patients' temperatures; Pupil Nurse Jones carries out all four-hourly mouth care and Staff Nurse Adams carries out all the dressings. This system is still widely used in the United Kingdom although it has been shown to be less effective than a patient allocation system, as well as causing a high degree of frustration among nurses (Bendall 1971; Briggs 1972). Task allocation has been perpetuated over the years as the traditional method. Tradition is a very comfortable thing which requires less thought and effort than new systems of thought.

Task allocation has a number of disadvantages. Firstly, it creates a job hierarchy. Jobs such as bathing or feeding helpless patients are considered to be of lowly status and are frequently allocated to junior learners or auxiliaries, while tasks of a more technical nature are considered to carry a high status and are allocated to senior nurses. Thus, activities which enable the nurse to spend time with a patient and to develop a personal relationship with him and which give her an excellent opportunity for direct observation of the patient, are seldom performed by a senior or qualified member of staff. Secondly, patient care becomes fragmented, and is seen as a series of unrelated tasks, each performed by a different nurse. Thirdly, task allocation tends to produce a rigid ward routine to which the nurses adhere, rather than to fit the routine to the patient's needs.

What is team nursing?

Here the nursing staff are organised into teams, each of which is led by a staff nurse or senior student nurse and looks after a group of patients. The team leader is responsible for planning the care of the patients for whom the team is responsible. She can use a patient-allocation system or a task-allocation system: more frequently it is the latter. Team nursing is better than task allocation in that the member of nurses caring for any one patient is reduced.

What is patient allocation?

With patient allocation, each nurse is allocated her own small group of patients. If staffing permits, one nurse can act as a 'runner' as well as being allocated fewer and/or lower-dependency patients of her own. She can then help other nurses with procedures such as bed-making and lifting, which require more than one nurse to carry out. Alternatively, two nurses can always work together when necessary, but the nurse to whom the patients have been allocated assumes responsibility for them and is accountable to the ward sister. Patient allocation does *not* mean that one nurse must carry out all the care for her patients, but it does mean that the nurse is responsible for the care being given.

Trained nurses can plan the nursing care for their own patients. Learners and inexperienced nurses will have to be supervised by Sister or Staff Nurse.

Different kinds of patient allocation   Patients can be allocated to nurses in several ways: for one span of duty only; for a longer period, eg. a week; or for the whole of a patient's stay in hospital. In this last instance the nurse would admit the patient, take an admission history, assess the patient, play a major part in defining his nursing problems, goals and nursing instructions and look after that patient whenever she is on duty throughout his stay in hospital.

The planning of care can also be arranged in several ways.

Firstly, it may be carried out by each shift of nurses on arrival for their span of duty; secondly, care for the next twenty-four hours may be planned by the responsible nurse whose plan is then followed by the other nurses caring for that patient at other times. If the care planning session is arranged during the shift overlap in the afternoon both the nurses concerned can be involved and any questions can be discussed as they arise. This system may also be extended to include long-term planning as well.

How to co-ordinate individual care with ward routines   As previously stated, one of the reasons why care planning is alien to the traditional pattern of nursing care in the UK is because the latter involves strict adherence to a rigid ward routine. Lelean (1974) said "adherence to routine could in part be due to procedure-centred nursing, thus the patient's care was never seen in total and her needs never fully met." The routine, in effect, became more important than the needs of the patient. Lelean suggested that one reason why certain tasks, such as hourly bedpans or two-hourly pressure area care, were not carried out as instructed by the sister was that nurses were so busy trying to keep up with the routine that anything which interrupted this was regarded as a nuisance and tended to be forgotten or put off until such time as it could be fitted in. Lelean suggested that this approach adversely affected patient care and that, therefore, in order to improve matters each patient should be treated according to his needs and not be made to fit into an inflexible ward system.

For example, if Mr Smith is the last patient on Student Nurse Black's list for bed baths, he may not have his bed bath until 11.00 or 11.30 a.m. This in itself may not matter. However, if Sister has also said that Mr Smith is to sit out in a chair for an hour in the morning before lunch and an hour in the afternoon, the morning 'hour' cannot then be fitted in. Getting all the bed baths done by mid-day becomes the important goal for Student Nurse Black and not the individual needs of the patients.

With patient allocation, routine can be replaced by a more flexible system which takes into account the patient's total needs. Of course, certain fixed times have to be taken into account such as four-hourly observations, meals etc., but since these will be done for the patient by his own nurse, she can plan the remainder of his day around these activities.

Advantages of patient allocation   *(a) It is more satisfying*   Task assignment has been shown to be a source of great frustration among nurses. The nurse feels that she is not caring for the patient as an individual but is performing a set of unrelated tasks with little functional reasoning behind them. Although both nurses and patients find patient allocation more satisfying, many wards still use task allocation. This kind of discrepancy creates a considerable amount of stress.

(b) It expands the rôle of the nurse   The use of patient allocation will mean re-defining the rôles of qualified nurses. The emphasis will be on their rôle as practitioners supervising the less experienced as well as teaching learners by example as they carry out bedside care.

Because the nurse is responsible for the care of her own patients the sister's rôle changes to that of a clinical supervisor, always available for consultation in case of difficulty but relieved of many interruptions. She therefore has more time to attend to the overall planning of her ward, to teach, to advise and to develop her own and her staff's clinical skills. She can refer many queries to the nurse to whom the patient in question has been allocated.

(c) It helps learners (as also does team nursing)   Patient allocation (and team nursing) will benefit learners. Both systems help them to gain confidence and experience in caring for patients, yet with supervision. Learners gain great satisfaction from knowing that they are playing a more important rôle in the planning as well as in the giving of care and that they have been made responsible for 'their' patients. At the same time they know they have support from more senior nurses and are not just left alone to cope unaided. Learners can also get to know their patients better, understand the precise reasons why particular aspects of care should be prescribed and performed, and have the opportunity of raising questions with senior nurses as well as with medical staff. Patient allocation (and team nursing) can also play a part in better preparation of the learners for their practical assessment by ensuring that the relevant experience has been gained.

(d) It leads to individual patient care   Although team nursing is a vast improvement on task allocation, to make nursing care truly individualised, patient allocation is necessary. The number of

patients allocated to each nurse will depend upon several factors:

> the seniority and experience of the nurse
> the nursing care needs of the patient
> the number of high-dependency patients in the ward
> the number of nurses on duty
> the total number of patients in the ward

When a patient is looked after by 'his own nurse' there is a stronger feeling of identity and security. He will develop a special relationship with that nurse and will always know to whom he can go for help. Ward activities revolve around the patients' needs rather than the ward routine. Because there is not the drive for all baths, dressings and beds to be completed by mid-day, other aspects of care, eg. two-hourly turns, can be carried out as prescribed, leaving other aspects of care until later. Thus the work is spaced out more evenly over the day and not concentrated between 8.00 a.m. and mid-day.

(e) It improves ward communication   Patient allocation improves written and verbal communication. A nurse who is responsible for the total care of a patient knows more about that patient and can give a better report on him than one who may nurse the patient for only a few minutes at a time. She is also able to report on all facets of her patient's condition, eg. state of skin, healing of wound, level of pain, mental state, etc. She is the best person, therefore, to write the Kardex report and to give verbal reports about the patient. The ward sister always knows whom to ask for information about a patient's condition and progress. Similarly, the medical staff can be taught to ask the patient's nurse for information instead of always asking Sister.

Naturally, Sister will retain overall responsibility. She will need to hear reports on all the patients and may perhaps have to give a general report on the patients in order to co-ordinate care with the doctors and para-medical staff. However, the introduction of care planning rounds and nurse-to-nurse handovers should be tried, as these provide the opportunity for more detailed discussion of the patients' needs and progress.

Summary

Patient allocation is an essential beginning to care planning. Nurses must see patients as individuals who require integrated care planned specifically for them, rather than being the recipients of a series of unrelated tasks peformed by different nurses. The ward sister has the most important rôle to play in achieving patient allocation. Once in use the benefits to both patients and staff will demonstrate that the change was worthwhile.

References

Bendall E. (1971) The learning process in student nurses. *Nursing Times,* **67** (43, 44), 169, occasional papers

Briggs A. (1972) *Report of the Committee on Nursing.* London: HMSO

Ethridge P. & Packard R. (1976) An innovative approach to measurement of quality through utilization of nursing care plans. *Journal of Nursing Administration,* Jan., 42-48

Lelean S. (1974) *Ready for Report, Nurse?* London: RCN

Matthews A. (1975) Patient allocation – a review. *Nursing Times,* **71** July 10, 17, 24, 31

Chapter 3

From Theory to Practice

Talking about and writing about Nursing Care Plans is all very well, but it is the translation of words into actions that is the real test of its value. There is an increasing number of hospitals where care planning and the nursing process are being tried. Much can be gained from the experience of others so this chapter describes our experience in the hope that others can benefit from our mistakes as well as our successes. All the ideas described in this book have been tried out by ward sisters and learners.

Nursing Care Plans based on the nursing process were introduced by us, in the first instance, at The London Hospital as part of a research project into the communication of nursing instructions and, secondly, as a project started by the qualified nurses on a psychogeriatric ward because they were keenly interested. These two projects created a great deal of interest in care plans and the nursing process, with the result that their use is being extended to other wards.

Nursing Care Plans: preparation and development

As a preliminary step, we looked at what other nurses were doing or had done in relation to using such plans and the nursing process. Furthermore, since doctors use a problem-orientated format their approach was also studied. The problem-orientated medical record was developed by Weed (1969) and its use has become widespread in the USA; it is also used by an increasing number of doctors in the United Kingdom. The literature provided both knowledge about the theories and concepts and practical examples of the formats used.

A research proposal was drawn up which included our first ideas about the format that might be used, and a timetable for the introduction of the Nursing Care Plans. This, in effect, established the goals and review data. A grant from the Regional Health Authority made it possible to undertake the project.

The nursing process became the framework within which the ideas and plans were developed, in conjunction with a model of nursing care (Fig. 1) developed by Hunt (1977). Basing the care plans on the nursing process meant that these had to have at least three components: one for assessment, one for the plan and one for the continuing record. The Nursing Care Plan consists therefore of a *nursing history,* a *Care Plan* and a *progress record.* In order for it to be acceptable to nurses on the wards the Nursing Care Plan had to contain certain factors. It had to be easy for nurses to use; it had to be large enough, and this meant A4 size; it had to be standardized and yet meet the needs of different wards; it had to fit the Kardex because the sisters at that time preferred to retain this system — this subsequently changed as the sisters decided to use ring folders, but the A4 size was retained.

The nursing history Because planning depends upon assessment, the design of the nursing history (Fig. 2) had to be the first task. Other nursing histories were considered but none were satisfactory. In order that it should reflect the ward needs, a ward sister was asked to draw up the first version, which was then tried out and changed where necessary. Suggestions for changes and improvements are particularly likely to occur with a new form because until it is in use, and has been used over a period of time, it is impossible to know whether it is the right format. Whenever possible, improvements suggested by the ward staff were incorporated into the nursing history. It is very important to use the suggestions made by the ward staff for not only does this demonstrate to the nurses that their ideas are of value but it also improves the form.

The Care Plan The second part of the Nursing Care Plan is the *Care Plan* itself (Fig. 3). A problem-orientated approach was taken which was very similar to that advocated by Mayers (1972). The identification of nursing problems is an essential step in the nursing process. Once the nursing problems have been listed, the nursing goals are established and the care is prescribed to reach the goals. As with the nursing history, the format of the Care Plan has been changed several times and the final version includes provision for discharge planning. This section is very essential and was included in the first instance in the nursing history when this was the only part of the Nursing Care Plan in use. Again, suggestions and ideas from ward staff were taken into account when changing the format.

The progress record   The final part of the Nursing Care Plan is the progress record (Fig. 4) and, again, several versions have been tried. The form now in use will serve either as a daily narrative-type record or as a problem-orientated one: that is, day-to-day progress can be recorded or a note can be written about progress with each problem. As the present progress record was brought into use before the Care Plan it is divided into two sections, one for 'progress' and the other for 'nursing instructions'. This preliminary step encouraged nurses to distinguish between instructions for care and reporting on care given, and as the form provided a special place for nursing instructions it meant that these were permanently recorded. However, this division becomes redundant once the Care Plan is in use since all instructions about nursing care are written on it.

Introducing Nursing Care Plans

Each part of the Nursing Care Plan was introduced separately. There were two main reasons for this decision: firstly, each element had to be evaluated and therefore it had to be possible to identify the changes resulting from each one. Secondly, it was better to be 'slow but sure', because neither the researchers nor the ward sisters knew enough about care planning or the nursing process when applied in the ward to plunge straight into full-scale implementation. This approach also helps to allay nurses' fears about change.

The nursing history form was introduced on one small ward in order to identify any changes needed in the format. Its use was then extended to another five wards and finally to five more. It is being used therefore on 10 large (27-bed) wards and one small metabolic unit. Of these wards, five are medical, four surgical and two are mixed.

The ward sisters introduced the nursing history at the pace they felt was appropriate, taking into account the ward workload and staffing. Teaching and any other help requested was provided by the researchers, who assumed responsibility for providing the necessary forms, Kardex holders and ring folders. While the nursing history was in use in only five wards the teaching was entirely ward based. However, now that so many wards are involved, preliminary teaching takes place in an Introductory Course, followed by back-up teaching in the wards. Once the nursing process becomes the basis for the educational programme, the teaching about the nursing history will be taken over by the tutorial staff. Other aids already provided to help nurses on an individual basis are a guide to completing the nursing history and a leaflet explaining in very simple terms the reasons for care planning using the nursing process (see Appendix II).

The new progress record was introduced soon after the nursing history form. This enabled the wards to change over completely to the A4 size of form. Again, sisters have been free to develop their use of the new form in their own way and at their own pace, which has provided much information about how it can be used and how the nurses feel. For example, it has become clear over a period of time that if the progress record is utilised as the only source of nursing instructions, especially when these are written in full for each shift, it becomes a much more useful document. Its use in this way has demonstrated, in particular, the value of having a detailed *permanent* record of nursing instructions, and has also provided a useful starting point for the development of the Care Plan. Obviously, when the Care Plan comes into use, the column for nursing instructions in the progress notes will no longer be necessary as these instructions will be listed in the Care Plan alongside the problems and goals.

The written Care Plan is the final and most concrete aspect of any systematic approach to nursing care. It was first tried by one ward. Nursing care plans were written and maintained for a group of patients over a period during which they were cared for by the Research Assistant. This demonstrated quite clearly that the method was both feasible and valuable. Two wards are now trying out the same type of Care Plans with considerable success. Again, the emphasis has been on ward-based teaching in order to introduce the nurses to a problem-orientated approach. Continuing help is then provided to supervise and advise on the writing of the Care Plans and to provide support and encouragement. Such teaching and supervision is essential, since most nurses think of nursing care as a series of tasks and investigations which result from the medical diagnosis and not in terms of nursing problems which are associated with but separate from this diagnosis.

Nursing Care Plans were introduced as part of the implementation of the nursing process research project. Such research is necessary if their use is to be based on accurate data, just as nursing should be based on the results of research. Because it is a research project the introduction of Nursing Care Plans may have taken longer than might otherwise have been the case. However, the research is providing factual data about the advantages and disadvantages of the new system and will enable any decision about extending it to be made on an informed and rational basis.

To illustrate how the introduction of Nursing Care Plans has affected different nurses within the hospital, three of them describe their experiences:*

THE RESEARCH ASSISTANT'S ACCOUNT

In January 1977 I applied for, and was appointed to the post of Research Assistant. The project upon which I was to work formed part of the continuing nursing research at the hospital, although it was a separate project in its own right.

A major part of the project was the introduction and use of individual Nursing Care Plans which would incorporate specific nursing instructions and also provide for more personalised nursing care. A move towards this concept had already been started with the introduction of individual work cards as a replacement for workbooks and worklists.

As the first step in the Nursing Care Plan experiment, we introduced a nursing history. The prototype had been designed by one of the ward sisters, but several revisions were needed before the layout satisfied the ward staff. It was essential to have a nursing history since without it nurses would have insufficient information on which to base their Care Plans. Initially, the nursing history was tried in four wards; later its use was extended to seven more. (As the form was A4 size, it was necessary to change the Kardex in these wards to this size; previously, a very small Kardex had been used.) Sisters and nurses were free to recommend changes and alterations in the format and whenever possible these were incorporated.

Two elements of a Nursing Care Plan were therefore in use: a nursing history sheet and progress notes. The next stage was to

*From *Rediscovering the Patient.* Nursing Times booklet. 30 November 1978.

introduce the Care Plan. We had become very convinced of the importance and value of the nursing process and so decided to introduce a problem-orientated Care Plan which would allow the nurses to record the patients' nursing problems, the goals for each problem, the care to be given to attain those goals and the final outcome so that we and they could see whether the goals were met. This meant that after completing the nursing history, the nurses had to identify the nursing problems or needs of that patient. Once they had done this we hoped to encourage the nurses to predict how long it should take for their nursing care to reach the goals and provide them, therefore, with the means to evaluate the care they were giving. If they said they would take a course of action for three days, regardless of who was on duty or in charge, when the three days were up, that particular nursing action would be evaluated to see if the goal had been reached.

Although this was what we wanted to introduce, we were not so idealistic as to think that it would be easy. For one thing, we learned right from the start not to use the phrase 'nursing process'. Some sisters had become antipathetic towards the nursing process after reading articles in the nursing press which they felt were too theoretical and impractical, so we used phrases like 'total patient care' or 'individual care plans' instead.

Nor did we presume that our success with the nursing history meant that we were going to have as much success with the next stage of our Care Plans. The staff of one ward started to use our problem-orientated approach and found no difficulty in writing problem lists but were reluctant to commit themselves to writing goals, probably because nurses do not like to commit themselves on paper, and also because it takes a great deal of learning to feel confident to do this. I demonstrated the practicability of writing care plans by caring for three weeks for a group of patients on one of the medical wards, using this approach. I found it perfectly feasible to write and maintain Nursing Care Plans, and the other nurses found them very useful. I also found that my nursing care of these patients had more positive direction. I was more aware of why I was carrying out care and what I was aiming at.

I found that care planning based on the nursing process allows nursing to work within its own boundaries rather than relying almost entirely on a medical diagnosis. It made nursing more exciting and interesting and enabled me to provide nursing care which was more relevant to the needs of the patients. I also found that many nurses will resist change, not only because they dislike the new idea, but just because it is a new idea. We are comfortable and complacent in our jobs. Of course I am generalising, but that was the attitude of many of the nurses with whom I came into contact. I was kept going, during the times when I became very frustrated, by those nurses and sisters who said "I'm not sure I agree with all this, but I will give it a try" and who, after trying it, then did not want to return to the old method, and by the memory of the student nurse on her first ward who, after I had explained what we were trying to do, said to me "But its so sensible. I don't understand why everyone doesn't do it this way".

A MEDICAL WARD SISTER'S ACCOUNT

When I was asked if I would like to introduce the taking of nursing admission histories from patients on my ward, I initially had some reservations. Having read articles on the nursing process, I was concerned that in a busy medical ward, at a busy time of the year (the winter months), we would not have enough time for the work that it appeared to involve. I was also concerned that because the majority of patients were admitted as emergencies it would be impractical to take the history immediately as on the whole such patients require urgent nursing attention. It was decided, therefore, that the history would be taken within the first 48 hours after admission.

The reasoning behind the history and ways of asking the appropriate questions was explained to all the staff by the Nursing Research Assistant, and a comprehensive written explanation was also provided. Initially, the learners listened while the Research Assistant took a history before they were allowed to take one themselves. Thereafter, a trained member of staff listened in but as we got used to the practice this ceased to be necessary. Now that nurses receive a lecture on the subject in the Introductory Course this initial ward lecture is no longer necessary, although nurses arriving on the ward have the procedure explained and read the written information.

Most of the staff took an immediate interest in the project and found that they enjoyed taking nursing histories. The time taken initially to complete the history was 15-30 minutes, but as we became more experienced it usually took less time than this, depending on how verbose the patient was and whether his history was simple or complicated.

By the end of the first week only two histories had not been taken, one patient being too ill and the other due for discharge. Sometimes histories were taken more than 48 hours after admission. Where a patient was too ill the history was taken from a relative or friend; this was sometimes a problem as some patients had neither. After a few weeks we found it possible to take the histories of patients admitted from the waiting list at the time of their admission. As we became more accustomed to the procedure we found also that we could take the history of emergency admissions at the same time as the rest of the admission procedure.

Taking histories has now become incorporated into the ward routine, and unless the ward is particularly busy or short of staff the histories are taken at or soon after admission.

The completed sheets are placed in the Kardex for anyone authorised to see. It has been said that the information contained in the nursing histories is also obtained by the doctor, but there is not always time to read the medical notes, nor do they always contain the information that the nurses need. I also feel that nurses should themselves obtain the details they need about their patients. In the past, one or two nurses would find out snippets of information, but they did not always pass these on; now such information is available for all the nurses to see, and can be up-dated if necessary.

No significant changes in nursing care have resulted from taking these histories. However, from the patient's point of view, I feel it is beneficial that every patient regardless of his age, condition, attitude, etc. should have a nurse asking him questions about himself for ten minutes or so as it makes him feel that the nurses are interested in him as an individual. Interestingly enough, no patient has refused to answer the questions.

Taking the history makes it possible to discover immediately if a patient has a particular problem which perhaps can be remedied there and then or the appropriate person notified. For example, a blind Frenchman, who spoke no English, was treated for his constipation soon after his admission because his daughter, when answering the history questions, said that he had been constipated for several days. I think it would have taken us several days to have discovered this without the history.

The occupational and physiotherapists are free to look at the mobility section and the social worker at the home and social section. This saves time because they do not have to ask a nurse what immediate help is needed, and it can also reduce the need to ask some preliminary questions.

An interesting section is that in which the patient is asked what he thinks is wrong with him. In several instances the patient has been found to have wrong information about his condition and we then had to decide, depending on the patient and his ability to comprehend, whether to inform him correctly ourselves or to tell the medical staff.

The learners enjoy asking the questions. They feel that they have more knowledge of the patient as an individual and have a special relationship with that person throughout his hospital stay. They feel the histories make them realise that patients are individual people and that this information both helped them in their practical work and would help them in future theoretical work, when they could think back to the patients they had nursed.

I feel that this new system is an improvement on the old, with interesting and helpful information obtained for the benefit of the patient. I will be happy to continue with this practice.

A PSYCHOGERIATIC WARD SISTER'S ACCOUNT

This acute admission ward with 18 beds (12 women, 6 men) caters for people over the age of 65 years. The majority of the patients suffer from functional illnesses such as depression, paranoid states, schizophrenia, manic reactions and personality disorders. A small percentage have organic illnesses such as acute confusional states. The average length of stay is from 4 to 6 weeks, although some patients stay longer for social reasons.

We thought that we needed Nursing Care Plans for several reasons. Firstly, we felt unclear over the rôle of the psychiatric nurse. We asked ourselves what nursing care we actually offered to each individual in our ward and what did this care achieve? Although intuitively we felt we were undertaking some form of care it was not systematic. Secondly, we were frustrated by the attitudes of our colleagues and our inability to make them aware of the rewards and problems in working with the elderly who are also mentally ill. Thirdly, we were aware of the lack of information in the Kardex system of record-keeping we were using. Fourthly, we felt that the medical diagnosis was inadequate as a basis for planning nursing care, and lastly, we felt that there was a need to attract skilled and interested nurses into the field of psychiatry in the elderly.

It was difficult to change the way we were looking at our nursing care. Many nurses felt that they already planned their care and knew the objectives of this care and what it achieved; however, anxiety was felt when it came to committing their analysis of patients' problems to paper and then to describing the specific nursing care to meet these problems. The difficulty we found in doing this demonstrated that our usual approach had been very general in application.

We worked through stages, beginning with a separate page for listing problems, intervention and planning for discharge. These were kept in individual folders with the daily progress notes. Eventually we achieved a practical system which included a nursing admission history, a problem/intervention record, and progress notes and discharge plan (Appendix I).

The admission history is completed by the nurse admitting the patient, thereby enabling the initial problems to be identified. The problem/intervention record is used daily at handover when group decisions are taken on plans, listing any new problems, deciding specific interventions and detailing problems resolved. We found that the ideal time to do this was during the overlap period of two hours when both morning and afternoon staff are on duty. The progress notes are written up during each span of duty. Details of behavioural patterns and care given are included, preferably avoiding the use of jargon. The discharge plan covers all follow up after discharge.

Since the Nursing Care Plans have been fully used I feel that the quality of patient care has improved. The nurses have a refreshing, positive approach to their work, they are questioning and more aware of the aims of their nursing care. They also now evaluate their care which in turn stimulates them to continue their questioning approach.

Introducing the Nursing Care Plans has not been easy. Enthusiasm from the trained staff, daily encouragement and reminders of our aims have been necessary. One problem has been the frequent changes of student nurses which has meant having to explain the approach to each newcomer. The positive side of this was that, without exception, all the student nurses showed interest and enthusiasm about Nursing Care Plans; in fact, without their support we would not have managed to establish the new system. Undoubtedly we still have a long way to go in planning our care, but we feel that we are at least beginning to bring a sense of professionalism to our work.

Summary

Theory cannot be translated into practice without some effort. It required not only the co-operation and participation of the nursing staff but also a considerable input of teaching time. At the present time the nursing process is still not taught to all learners so the teaching of care planning on the wards has to include the basic concepts as well as their practical application. Obviously the best approach is where the school and wards complement and reinforce each other's teaching. Positive encouragement from administration is also necessary. It is vital that Nursing Care Plans become accepted as an integral part of nursing care when practised rather than as something taught in school but too impractical or theoretical for day to day use. Their use as a continuing, everyday tool in the wards is essential.

Implementation on a wider scale demands a more formal in-service education programme. Each course must include an introduction to the theoretical background, to the uses which can be made of the theories and to the practicality of the system they, the nurses, will be using. Practice must based on logical ideas and then put into practice. Most important, nursing officers and teaching staff must listen to what the ward sisters and staff are saying. They must be aware of the fears and anxieties (real or imagined) about adopting a new way of planning nursing care and must include the ideas and thoughts of the staff on the wards when introducing any changes.

References

Mayers M. (1972) *A Systematic Approach to Nursing Care Plans*. New York: Appleton-Century-Crofts
Weed L. (1969) *Medical Records, Medical Education and Patient Care*. Cleveland: Case Western Reserve University

The Four Stages of Nursing Care Plans

In Section I we took an overall look at care planning, followed by a discussion of the relationship between care planning and methods of organising patient care, and we described our experience at The London Hospital. Now we turn to look in depth at care planning. Each of the four stages is discussed in turn beginning with assessment and ending with evaluation. We have drawn throughout on our own experiences, and the examples quoted are real; they are not perfect because we were, and still are, learning how to use care planning as a tool for better patient care.

What are Nursing Care Plans?

Nursing Care Plans are written for individual patients and are a practical way of putting the nursing process to work. They are not the same thing as the nursing process, although there is a definite relationship between the activity of producing Nursing Care Plans and the philosophy of the nursing process. Producing a Nursing Care Plan involves assessing the patient's needs and planning appropriate care. The nursing care can then be given, or modified and adapted as necessary, using the written record called the Nursing Care Plan; furthermore, care given can subsequently be evaluated. A Nursing Care Plan is, therefore, a practical tool which helps nurses to give individualised care to patients.

A Nursing Care Plan has four purposes. It provides an assessment of the patient's needs; details of the planned care; a description of how this was implemented, and an evaluation of the outcomes for the patient. These steps correspond to the four stages of the nursing process. Learning about Nursing Care Plans, and gaining practice in their use, should help nurses towards a clearer understanding of the principles of the nursing process.

39

It is important that readers should understand the terminology which has been used throughout the book, to avoid the danger of confusion. When we talk about *Nursing Care Plans,* (ie. capital initial letters and preceded by Nursing) we mean all the paperwork which is needed to put the nursing process to work, including the patient's history, his progress notes, and the planned programme of patient care itself.

However, when we speak of the whole process of decision-making and recording which is necessary in order to produce a Nursing Care Plan, we have termed this activity *care planning* (ie. without 'nursing' and without capital initials). On occasion, particularly in Chapters 3 and 5, we will need to refer to that part of the whole Nursing Care Plan which contains just the written list of the patient's problems, and corresponding actions and goals. We have called this document the *Care Plan,* but wherever we have used this phrase we have differentiated it from the whole Nursing Care Plan.

Chapter 4

Assessment

This chapter is about the first step in care planning — assessment
— without which effective care planning is impossible. It
includes:

> collecting the information;
> interpreting the information; and
> defining the patient's nursing problems.

1 Collecting the information

What kind of information is needed?   All of the relevant information about the patient's past health, present health problems,
social history, habits of daily living, likes and dislikes, the nurses'
observations about the patient and a general overview of his
condition should be collected. This information is obtained both
from the patient and from other sources such as his notes and his
relatives, to enable care to planned and given for the patient
which is related to his particular needs.

Why do we need a nursing history?   The existing ways in which
nurses obtain and record information from their patients are
usually rather haphazard. There are various reasons why this
may be so. Firstly, nurses are not taught how to ask relevant
questions or how to use the answers or comments made by
patients to their greatest advantage. Secondly, some nurses are
less skilled at obtaining information from patients than others. In
the absence of training and structured history sheets, the quality
of their assessment is likely to be extremely variable. Thirdly,
information may or may not be passed on to the sister or nurse in
charge of the ward, who in turn may or may not decide to record
it. Fourthly, there is a rarely any place where detailed information about patients can be recorded in a systematic, orderly
fashion so that it is readily available.

What are the benefits of taking a nursing history? The benefits of taking a nursing history have been recognised by many writers. For example, Mayers (1978) states that a nursing history obtained from a patient by a nurse has several beneficial results. The most obvious is that the information gained gives the responsible nurse the necessary data for making a nursing diagnosis, ie. a list of the patient's problems which fall within the independent jurisdiction of nursing. She then lists the following additional benefits.

1 It is the commencement of the nurse-patient relationship. The patient sees the nurse as someone who cares about him as an individual, and it increases his feelings of trust in the nurse.
2 It stimulates the patient to become involved in his care which can lead to his increased co-operation regarding his treatment.
3 It strengthens the nurse's commitment. By talking to her patient and learning something about his habits, likes and dislikes, the nurse sees him in a more personal light and not just as a sick person who, accorded a diagnosis, should conform to signs, symptoms and care in a predictable way.
4 It saves time and energy. A nursing history enables problems to be identified, can prevent or alleviate problems and provides the nurse with information for forward planning.

Why not use the medical history? A nursing history is needed even though a medical history has been obtained. A nursing history focuses on finding out about the patient and his family as a basis for planning *nursing* care and determining the amount and type of *nursing* assistance he will need, whereas a medical history is taken to determine whether pathology is present as a basis for planning medical care and treatment. The use of a nursing history, therefore, enables a nurse to collect information relevant to the nursing needs of the patient, evaluate that information and identify the patient's nursing problems. Then the nursing care can be planned and implemented.

What form should a nursing history take? The aim is to produce a nursing history which will provide nurses with the information they need to identify the patient's nursing problems and needs, and be acceptable to the nurse. It is essential that the nursing history can be completed within a reasonable length of time in relation to the workload and staffing of the clinical setting.

There is a number of theoretical frameworks within which nursing histories have been designed, although this can mean that there is too much emphasis on the theory. Our approach to designing a form was very pragmatic. It included asking a ward sister to state what information she needed to know and wished to have recorded, and studying a large number of nursing histories produced by other people as well as looking at the theoretical concepts which could be used.

In the end, three different approaches were used. Firstly, that patients' nursing problems and needs could be physiological, psychological, emotional, environmental or social. Secondly, that nursing care should aim to retain and/or promote the patient's own pattern of daily living. Thirdly, that patients' nursing problems include both those stated or recognised by the patient and those recognised only by the nurse in the first instance.

Our nursing history includes, therefore:

> health information, including current diagnosis and operation, past and present health problems, and allergies (Fig. 7).
> social information such as occupation, dependents, housing, etc. (Fig. 8).
> the patient's perception of the reason for his admission (Fig. 9).
> the patient's description of his usual pattern of daily living activities such as sleep, diet, bowel habits, etc. (Fig. 10).
> the patient's and/or the nurse's description of the patient's condition including hearing, vision, mobility, etc. (Fig 11).

Because our nursing history record forms part of the ward record system, space is included also (Fig. 12) for essential reference information such as address, next of kin, etc. This not only made the nursing history more useful but also eliminated the need for any transcribing of such information to or from other records.

Nursing histories are essential for the systematic recording of relevant information about a patient. A conceptual framework is essential to provide coherence. However, the design of the nursing history is very important. The nursing staff must decide what they want from a nursing history before one can be designed

---

Diagnosis _____

_____

_____

_____

Operations on present admission   date performed

_____

_____

_____

_____

Past medical history/operations _____

_____

_____

_____

_____

_____

Allergies_____

History of present complaint _____

_____

_____

_____

Other current health problems_____

Fig. 7   The nursing history: health information

which will meet their needs since if it is not acceptable to them they will not use it. However, the needs of the organisation must also be considered, and this usually means some degree of standardisation. So, compromise and consensus become key words to ensure acceptability and availability.

How should a nursing history be taken?   The nursing history should be completed within a fairly short time following the patient's admission, although not necessarily on admission, or all at one time. Information may be added as and when it becomes available. However, information which is a record of the nurse's assessment or observation of the patient should not be altered since this information about the patient (at the time of interview)

SOCIAL HISTORY   Occupation_____

Children_____

Other dependants_____

HOUSING (House, flat – which floor, stairs,

lives alone, shares, bathroom/toilet)_____

_____

_____

_____

_____

Other problems at home?_____

_____

Visiting problems?   Yes   No

If Yes, describe:_____

Care at home: Details/Names

Community Nurse   _____

Social Worker   _____

Social Services   _____

(Please state   _____

specific service)   _____

G.P. (Name)   _____

_____

_____

_____

Fig. 8   The nursing history: social information

What *patient* says is the reason for admission_____

_____

_____

_____

_____

Fig. 9   The nursing history: the patient's perception

provides a baseline for later assessment of the patient's progress
— or his decline.

Most information is obtained by interviewing the patient,

DAILY LIVING

<u>DIET</u>

Special _____

Food or drink dislikes: _____

_____

Appetite: Good   Poor

Remarks _____

_____

<u>SLEEP</u> How many hours usually? _____

Sedation _____

Other comments _____

ELIMINATION

BOWELS: Any problems: Yes   No

If Yes, describe _____

_____

How often are bowels opened? _____

_____

Any medication? _____

URINARY: No problems   Incontinence

                      Nocturia   Dysuria

                      Frequency   Urgency

Remarks _____

_____

FEMALE PATIENTS – MENSTRUATION

     Regular   Irregular

     Amenorrhoea   Dysmenorrhoea

     Post-Menopausal   Taking the Pill

Next period due _____

Will need: ST's   Tampons

Remarks _____

Fig. 10   The nursing history: the activities of daily living

although some can be obtained from the patient's relatives, or by
direct observation of the patient. If the patient is not well enough
to give the information it must be obtained entirely from the

relatives and by direct observation by the nurse. Naturally, in an emergency the nurse concentrates solely on life-saving action and only obtains the information needed in order to take that action.

The way in which the information is obtained is very important. Questions should be concise and to the point and only one question should be asked at a time, eg. "Do you have any children?" — "Do you have other dependants?" rather than "Do you have any children or dependants?" Lay terms should be used as far as possible so that the patient can understand the questions, but it is important also not to talk down to the patient. Example: "Do you have to get up in the night to pass water?" rather than "Do you suffer from nocturia?" Questions should be asked in a way which obtains an answer which is more than just 'yes' or 'no', eg. "How do you feel today?" will elicit more information from the patient than "Do you feel all right today?" Questions should be worded so that they do not bias the patient's answer, eg. "Do you feel nauseated as well?" may make the patient think that the nurse expects him to feel nauseated.

When conducting an interview to obtain information from the patient on admission it is important to have the right approach and attitude. Remember that the patient is probably anxious, nervous and unwell. The nurse must give her full attention to the patient. She must also be prepared to sit and listen, and, while not restricting his answers, to keep the interview progressing. Other patients should not be able to overhear the answers. Every effort should be made to ensure peace and quiet, and freedom from interruptions. The nurse must at least appear unhurried, since, if the patient feels that the nurse is busy and wants to get on with other activities, he may well try to hurry through his answers.

Before beginning the interview the nurse must explain to the patient why she is asking all the questions. She must then listen carefully to the responses given by the patient and make sure that what she records on the nursing history form is accurate and meaningful. Nurses also need to learn to recognise non-verbal cues which often express a more honest account of what the patient feels, and so are very important bits of information.

Information should also be as free from judgmental phrases such as 'good' or 'bad' as possible. What is good to one nurse may not be good to another.

Fig. 11   The nursing history: the patient's appearance and condition

HEARING	Right:	Good
	Left:	Good
Hearing Aid?	Yes	No
Remarks_____		
VISION	Right:	Good
	Left:	Good
	Glasses	
Remarks_____		

PROSTHESIS/APPLIANCE/AIDS

Type(s)_____

_____

Any help needed?   Yes

MOBILITY   Fully mobile?

If no – needs help with:

Walking	Standing
Washing	Bathing
In/Out of bed	In/Out of chair

_____

_____

ORAL

Any problems with mouth or teeth?

If Yes, describe_____

Wears dentures?   Yes   No

_____

Any problems with dentures?_____

_____

_____

Any crowns?_____

Who takes the nursing history?   Both qualified nurses and learners can be taught how to interview a patient to obtain admission information. A written guide to filling in the nursing history is a useful aid to help nursing staff on the ward (Appendix II).

Teaching is necessary. In the early stages, particularly if the nursing history is only in use on some wards, it has to be ward based. However, it is more economical in terms of time and effort

		NURSES OBSERVATIONS		
or	Deaf			
or	Deaf	**ATTITUDE**		
		Anxious	Withdrawn	Distressed
		Remarks – (If particular problem please try and state reason e.g.		
or	Blind	anxious about operation/or being in hospital etc.		
or	Blind			
ntact Lenses				
		GENERAL APPEARANCE		
		Normal	Obese	
No		Dehydrated	Thin	
Yes	No	Acutely ill	Emaciated	
		Remarks		
Dressing				
Feeding				
Other		**SKIN**		
		Satisfactory	Broken areas	
		Dehydrated	Rash	
		Oedematous	Jaundiced	
		Describe		
Yes	No			
Upper	Lower	**LEVEL OF CONCIOUSNESS**		
		Orientated	Semi-conscious	
		Confused	Unconscious	
		Remarks		

to incorporate teaching about history taking and assessment into the training programme, both basic and post-basic, and also into the in-service education programme for trained staff. Even then, back up teaching and supervision will still be needed, as for all nursing skills.

Other sources of information   Completion of the nursing history is not the only source of information about the patient. There are

Record Number_____
PATIENT LABEL
Name_____
Address_____
_____
_____
_____
Date of Birth_____ Age_____
Date of Admission_____ Time_____
Type: Emergency   Planned
Transfer from_____
Marital status_____ Religion_____
Next of Kin (Name)_____
Relationship to Patient_____
Address_____
_____
_____
Tel. No(s)_____
_____
Speech difficulty/language barrier
Consultant_____
House Officer_____

Fig. 12   The nursing history: reference information

a number of other sources which the nurse may use either to provide new information or to check on that already obtained from the patient. Firstly, there is the nurse's own knowledge. Clearly this knowledge base can add considerably to the nurse's assessment of the patient's condition through her understanding of the underlying anatomy and physiology, the way humans respond to stress, the effect of the patient's illness on the body systems, etc. Secondly, there is the 'expert' knowledge which the nurse seeks in order to provide information that she lacks. Such knowledge could come from the patient's medical notes, from more experienced and knowledgeable colleagues both nursing, medical and para-medical, or from reference books and other published material. Finally, information about the patient can be obtained from those who know him well, such as friends and relatives. Such sources are particularly important if the patient is either too ill or unable to give the nurse any information himself.

Naturally, not all these sources have to be tapped for every nursing problem or every patient, nor even when it is necessary need such information be obtained immediately, unless such immediacy is demanded by the urgency of the patient's needs. Whenever possible, nurses should be encouraged to seek additional information. When they have done so, the information must be welcomed and used by the senior members of staff. Effort should not go unrewarded because if it does, it becomes less and less likely that such effort will be made.

It is important that nurses should recognise that they have a responsibility to ensure that their knowledge represents the most up-to-date information available on the nursing problem in question. Continuing education and up-dating is an obligation, not a luxury. Patients deserve and should get the most knowledgeable care.

2 Interpreting the information

Putting the pieces together: once the admission information is collected the nurse should re-read it to try to find relationships between pieces of information. For example, in our first experiments using nursing histories the ward sister chose to try one out with a patient who was reported by the night nurse as having slept only for about four hours: "Could Sister please have a word with the House Officer and get some medication written up?" When asked by the ward sister how many hours a night she usually slept, the patient replied cheerfully "Oh, about four or five". Further questioning elicited that this had been her sleep pattern for many years, that she was not bothered by not sleeping much, and that she was quite happy to leave things as they were. Since she was happy there was no reason to interfere and in fact, giving her sedation would have been wrong because it would have upset her normal pattern of sleep quite unnecessarily. Obviously, if she had been unhappy with her sleep pattern, her difficulty in getting enough sleep would then have been identified as a nursing problem and the appropriate care planned.

Putting the information together is rather like doing a jigsaw puzzle: the more pieces that are fitted together, the more complete the picture. Junior nurses, learners and the inexperienced must therefore be helped by senior nurses to do this and senior nurses must demonstrate by example how the information can be used. One way of doing this is to 'talk through' all the decisions that they make about the nursing care of patients so that their reasons for making the decision can be passed on to the other members of the nursing team. Furthermore, the sisters can show the value they place on care planning by allocating time for it, by requiring their nurses to write care plans and by showing interest and enthusiasm in the care planning that the nurses undertake.

3 Identifying a patient's nursing problems

What is a nursing problem? A patient's nursing problem is identified from the acquisition or interpretation of information and is, therefore, anything of concern to either patient or nurse which can be helped, solved or ameliorated by specific nursing actions. By identifying a nursing problem the nurse has determined that there is a need for nursing care. We call them patients' nursing problems although others use different terms such as needs, concerns, nursing diagnosis.

Not all diseases or disabilities indicate a need for nursing intervention. If a patient has lost the use of his right hand but has learned to use his left hand to carry out his normal activities, there is then no need for intervention by nurses because no real problem is identified. If, however, the patient loses the use of one arm and is unable to perform his normal daily activities, there is then a need for nursing intervention because a patient's nursing problem has been identified.

---

1. Chest pain caused by angina. She is sweating, has a tachycardia and says she is in pain.

2. Anxiety caused by hospitalisation and not really understanding why she has been admitted. She is over-talkative and is constantly wringing her hands.

Fig. 13 Statement of a patient's nursing problem (an elderly woman with angina)

The statement of the patient's nursing problem should be clear, concise and should identify all the factors relating to the problem. Medically-determined problems may also be included if there are specific nursing actions which need to be taken to help the patient overcome them (see Fig. 13). Many nursing problems are independent of medical ones, even when related to the medical diagnosis.

How to write out a nursing problem   A full statement of a patient's nursing problem (Fig. 13) should include:

> identification of the problem
> identification of the cause of the problem (if known)
> identification of how the patient is behaving in relation to the problem.

However, in practice giving such detail is not always feasible and only identification of the nursing problem may be included.

The problems which are identified must be ones which can be influenced by nursing action. By including the cause of the problem as well as how the patient is behaving in relation to the problem; all nurses become aware of the cause-effect relationship between problems and behaviour. Causation is one of four types: physiological, psychological, social or economic. Identifying the cause is very important since the same problem may have more than one cause. For example, chest pain may be caused by angina, as quoted, but it could also be due to a chest infection, to trauma, to surgery, to shingles or to cancer. Knowledge of the cause enables nurses to plan appropriate care and to know what to look for in order to note those changes which show whether or not the problem is being solved.

Listing the problems – identifying priorities   Problems should be listed as far as possible in terms of priority. This is not always feasible because a problem may be listed at first as having low priority and can then achieve a high priority if the condition of the patient changes. Acute problems should be listed first, followed by long-term ones, so that nurses are reminded of them and preventive action can be taken. If, for example, during an admission interview the nurse learns that the patient is bedridden and observes that he is thin and has a dry dehydrated skin, the nurse would then identify *possible pressure sores* as a problem and add this to the list of the patient's nursing problems. In this way, pressure area care becomes a high priority as soon as the patient is admitted and not after his skin begins to go red or to break down. Of course, pressure area care would included in routine nursing care but identified in this way it becomes a priority and a special need for that patient. Also, by including the dry, dehydrated skin as part of the patient's problem, pressure area care would also be linked with giving fluids to deal with the dehydration.

The order in which problems are listed needs some discussion, because while they should be listed in terms of priority for the patient and the nursing care carried out according to these priorities, at present this is often not the case. Instead, most nursing care is carried out with nurses' priorities in mind, for example, the need for all baths, beds and dressings to be done before noon. However, because each nurse can easily have her own notions about what is most important it is a good idea for each ward or unit to decide on its criteria for establishing priorities. This is best done by using a particular model of nursing such as one of those mentioned in Chapter 8.

Summary

Assessment is much more than just taking a nursing history. Firstly, such a history has to be complemented by other information, particularly when the patient cannot answer questions himself. Secondly, the information *has* to be used. It is pointless to spend time obtaining information which nobody looks at and which is not utilised constructively. To be of value it must be used to identify the patient's nursing problems.

References

Crow J. (1977) The nursing process – 2: how and why to take a nursing history. *Nursing Times,* **73** (June 23), 950-957

Lewis L. (1970) *Planning Patient Care.* Dubuque, USA: Wm. Brown

Maslow A. (1962) *Toward a Psychology of Being.* Princeton, N.J.: Van Nostrand

Mayers M. (1978) *A Systematic Approach to Nursing Care Plans.* New York: Appleton-Century-Crofts

McCain R. (1965) Nursing by assessment – not intuition. *American Journal of Nursing,* April, 82-84

Chapter 5

Planning

The next step in care planning is to decide what nursing care a patient will need: this stage is called planning. The information obtained by the nurse during the admission interview, together with her observations and assessment, will enable her to identify the patient's nursing problems; these are then included on the care plan, with life-threatening problems listed and dealt with first, continuing, less urgent problems second, and possible problems third. Once the nursing problems have been listed the nurse can then plan the necessary nursing care.
Planning (Fig. 14) includes:

> setting the goal (or expected outcome) for each problem;
> deciding what nursing care will meet the stated goals and writing the appropriate instructions; and
> deciding when to review or evaluate each problem to see if the goal is being achieved.

1 Setting the goals

Goals are set for every nursing problem (Fig. 15). The problem list is therefore the starting point for this stage of care planning and is obtained from the nurses's

> interpretation of stated facts (received verbally when taking the nursing history),
> observation of the patient's physical condition (eg. degree of mobility, condition of skin over pressure areas, physical signs),
> interpretation of any non-verbal information (eg. attitude, mood), and
> assessment of information from other sources.

All this information is utilised by the nurse to formulate her Care Plans.

Formal identification of patients' nursing problems is rarely carried out at the present time. It is a new approach but one which can soon be learned, and the nurses' ability to identify problems and become proficient in this new skill improves with practice and experience.

Whenever or wherever a problem has been defined, a goal then needs to be set, in writing, which specifies the solution (or alleviation) it is hoped will be achieved. When this is done all the nurses, no matter which span of duty they are working, will understand what the prescribed nursing care is expected to achieve. Furthermore, the patient can also have the same knowledge and so become more involved in his own care. Goal-setting also means that nurses can evaluate the effectiveness of their actions by comparing the result with the goal, thereby identifying

DATE	NO	PATIENT'S NURSING NEEDS/PROBLEMS AND CAUSES OF PROBLEMS (N B Physiological, Psychological, Social and Family problems)	
12.3.80	3	Possible pressure sores due to poor skin – because of arthritis, previous radiotherapy, general immobility.	Healthy,

Fig. 14   Care Plan: problem, goal, instructions, review date

whether or not it has been successfully achieved. Without a written goal for each nursing problem, nursing care cannot be evaluated, so there is a continuing risk that care will be ineffective (or less effective than it should be). To be measurable goals have to be stated in quantifiable terms, that is written as a behavioural response of the patient, a verbal response, an observation or assessment by the nurse, or as a physiological measurement (Fig. 16).

The need for patient-centred goals Goals should be patient-centred. They should be written in terms of what the patient will be able to do when the problem is solved and not what the nurse will do. Goals should be stated in as precise terms as possible so

GOALS	NURSING INSTRUCTIONS	REVIEW ON/BY	DATE RESOLVED
intact skin	(a) Change position every 2 hours; straighten sheets; remove crumbs, if any; use draw sheets. 2 nurses to turn patient.	Once daily	
	(b) Personal hygiene — keep skin clean & dry. Daily bed bath with assistance. Don't forget hair & nails.	Daily	
	(c) Encourage nourishing diet with adequate protein and at least 2 litres fluid	14·3·80 15·3·80	

PATIENT'S NURSING PROBLEMS	GOALS
Acute back pain	Relief of pain
Constipation due to enforced bed rest	Usual, once daily, bowel action
Lack of interest in diet	Interest to be regained – meals eaten, patient says has enjoyed them
Has had previous deep vein thrombosis and chest infection	Prevention of recurrence during this admission

Fig. 15   Examples of problems and goals

that they are not open to different interpretations by other nurses. To establish the goal relating to a problem the nurse must decide, firstly, what leads her to recognise that the patient has a problem and, secondly, how she would expect the patient to respond, or what she might expect to see which will convince her that the problem has been solved. The information on which the nurse's decision is made and goals are formulated, will come from three main sources:

what the patient tells the nurse about his symptoms;
how the patient behaves or acts; and
clinical observation by the nurse of physical signs.

Finally, goals should be positive, that is, they should be stated wherever possible in terms of how the patient will respond or behave rather than how he will not. The intervention selected by

GOAL		TYPE OF RESPONSE	
No pain	as shown by	patient sitting up and talking	(behavioural)
		patient says his pain has gone	(verbal)
		colour normal	(observational)
		pulse now 88 beats per minute	(physiological)

Fig. 16   Types of responses for goals

the nurse should, if practicable, actively involve the patient. A good start in goal setting is to find out from the patient what he hopes the outcome of any problem will be; his nursing care then becomes meaningful rather than an unrelated series of actions. Nurse and patient working in co-operation in this way make the care more effective.

2 Deciding upon nursing instructions to achieve these goals

Nursing instructions are a list of the actions which the nurse prescribes in order to achieve the stated goal. These instructions should always be written. Nursing instructions will be aimed at anticipating a possible problem and preventing it from becoming an actual problem. The action or instruction prescribed is specific to that patient and that problem. Senior nurses use their knowledge, experience and expertise to decide what to prescribe, but junior nurses will obviously need the help of their seniors in deciding which actions are appropriate. The nurse must select that action which will best meet the patient's need. On some Care Plans the nurse may list several possible nursing actions for each problem; this is useful since it makes the nurse aware that there may be more than just *one* action to reach the goal, and also ensures that an alternative is readily available.

Nursing instructions must:

be based upon sound, scientific principles;
be specific and clear so that no matter which nurse is carrying out the care, she will interpret each instruction in the same way;
be realistic in terms of the nursing time and skill available to perform the care, and
prescribe care which will achieve the stated goal.

The nursing actions which are most likely to succeed will be soundly based upon scientific principles, realistic, work towards an established goal and planned with, and explained to, the patient so that he understands not only that something is being done but also why it is being done. Obviously, new ideas should, and must, be tried out — nursing care should be innovative. As long as the proposed nursing procedure is safe there is no reason why it should not be tried, provided that it is evaluated to see if (*a*) it reaches its goal and (*b*) whether it does so more, or less, effectively than the action it replaced.

DATE	NO	PATIENT'S NURSING NEEDS/PROBLEMS AND CAUSES OF PROBLEMS (N B Physiological, Psychological, Social and Family problems)	
16.3.80	1	Dehydration due to inadequate fluid intake, as seen by:	
		dry, dehydrated skin	(a) Adequate
		dry lips, coated tongue	(b) Moist
		decreased urinary output	(c) Urinary Least 2000
		Concentrated urine	(d) Urine (specific gra
		Constipation	(e) Daily

Fig. 17   Care Plan: replacing the instruction 'encourage fluids'

Instructions must be specific and explicit   The importance of specificity must be stressed, since this ensures that the patient receives the intended care which the nurse prescribed. Research[1,2] has shown that if instructions are too generalised they will be interpreted in many different ways. Consequently, one nurse's interpretation of an instruction, eg. 'mobilise' or 'up and about', may be totally different from another nurse's interpretation of the same instruction, and from that of the nurse who gave it.

For example, 'encourage fluids' is an instruction which is used frequently. What does it mean? It certainly does not indicate to

GOALS	NURSING INSTRUCTIONS	REVIEW ON/BY	DATE RESOLVED
hydration	To have at least 3000 ml. daily	Daily	
	0800 - 1600 — 1500 ml.	1400 hrs	
	1600 - 2200 — 1000 ml.	2000 hrs	
	2200 - 0800 — 500 ml.	0700 hrs	
	Sit patient well up before giving her her drink. Offer drinks hourly. Prefers tea, lemon, iced water. DOES NOT LIKE COFFEE.		
lips & tongue	Mouth care 4-hourly with mouthwash tablets and lemon glycerine to lips		
output of at ml. per day	Observe and record output. Report inadequate output.	Daily	
concentration with 1000 - 1010	Test urine for specific gravity; report abnormal findings		
bowel action	Record bowel action. Add bran to breakfast cereal. Encourage to eat fruit. Give aperient, as prescribed.	Daily	

the nurse how much fluid to give a patient, when to give it, what sort of fluid he needs, how often to give fluids or in what way they should be given. The result is that the fluid intake of the patient often varies greatly from one day to the next. When the instruction is specific (Fig. 17) the patient's intake fluctuates much less.

In many cases the nurse will prescribe nursing care which falls entirely within her own sphere of responsibility. However, there will be times when this is not so, when she has to obtain instructions from, or in consultation with, other members of the health care team. Again, these instructions should be precise and detailed enough to ensure they are implemented as intended.

3 When should the progress of a patient's nursing problem be reviewed or evaluated?

In order that the effectiveness of nursing care can be measured, nurses must state AT THE SAME TIME AS THEY GIVE THE INSTRUCTIONS how soon the nursing care should be reviewed in order to assess whether it is achieving the stated goal. The time limits set for reviewing a goal will vary. What is important is that such time limits be both specific to each goal, and realistic (Fig. 18).

With precise time limits such as those illustrated, all nurses work to the same time scale. In the case of analgesia given for pain, the nurse has decided to wait to see if the drug is acting and, if so, to reassess after $3\frac{3}{4}$ hours to see whether the pain has been relieved until the next dose is due. If at either of those times the goal had not been reached, the nurse would then take appropriate action, which may mean informing the medical staff that the analgesia is not having the desired effect, or implementing some nursing care already prescribed for this problem.

By setting a specific date or time for the evaluation of nursing actions, all nurses will know not only what the goals are but the anticipated time limit for their achievement. This ensures that failure of any nursing action to meet the desired goals will be noted, the need for change recognised and the necessary change made.

The ward sister's rôle in planning care   Most nurses would say that it is sister's responsibility to plan care, but the Salmon report on nursing (1969) listed the twelve rôles of the ward sister yet planning care was not mentioned. Who is responsible, therefore, for planning care? In patient allocation, each nurse is meant to plan the care of her patients. In team nursing it is the team leader. This question of responsibility is important and will become increasingly more so. In care planning there is an obvious need to re-define certain traditional rôles. The rôle of the ward sister takes on a new dimension: rather than having added burdens put upon her by these care plans, her rôle is changed so that some of her present tasks and responsibilities are delegated elsewhere while, at the same time, new responsibilities are given to her. The ward sister becomes a clinical expert on matters which need her skill and experience. She can leave nurses, depending on their ability and seniority, to plan the care for their patients but at the same time she makes herself available to act as a resource person and to guide junior learners in care planning. For example, with patient allocation the ward sister no longer has the task of writing

PATIENT'S NURSING PROBLEM	GOALS	REVIEW ON/BY
14.3.80		
Pain from laparotomy incision as seen by: – raised pulse	– pulse down to within 70–90 beats/minute	30 minutes
– sweating	– patient no longer sweating	2 hourly
– restlessness	– quiet and peaceful	2 hourly
– patient complaining of pain	– patient says he is pain free	30 mins & $3\frac{3}{4}$ hours after injection

Fig. 18   Care Plan: review date/time

the Kardex on her own. Instead, each nurse writes the progress notes for her patients under the ward sister's guidance. This way, the ward sister can assist learners to acquire this important skill early on during their training and under supervision. Consultants' ward rounds take on a new dimension for the nurse whose patient is under discussion, as she joins the round in order that she can give first hand information.

The nurses' rôle in planning care   The nurses' rôle also changes. Rather than just following instructions because sister has given them, the learner plays a part in deciding the instructions under supervision. She also is responsible for keeping the Care Plan up to date, communicating the plan, the patient's progress, any instructions and changes in the patient's condition to sister and the medical staff. (The subject of ward communication will be discussed in greater detail in the next chapter.)

There has been a great deal of discussion recently about what grades of staff should take part in the assessment and planning stages of the nursing process. Some senior nurses are concerned that students and pupils are not equipped to assess patients' needs and plan care, and many feel that learners should not take admission histories. Yet, with proper teaching, supervision, guidance and follow-up even the most junior learner can be taught these nursing skills as they are taught many others. The rôle of the clinical teacher is extended in teaching learners these new skills. Junior learners need guidance in interpreting information received from an admission history and from their observations of the patient. One way to encourage this is for junior nurses to re-read the history they have taken and the observations they have made and put an asterisk (*) next to any item on the history sheet which seems important to them or which could constitute a patient/nursing problem. This could be the initial first step in teaching nurses how to plan care from information and observation. One ward sister known to the authors who has been using admission histories for some time asks one of the nurses to present an assessment of her new patient at the ward report after having taken a history. Planning is then carried out with that nurse as well as with the others present. With a little thought and imagination a good ward sister can create many such opportunities to assist her nurses to plan care and to acquire sound clinical judgment.

Summary

Planning begins with patients' nursing problems. When these have been listed goals can then be set and instructions given for nursing care to meet these goals. It is important, also, to establish the time limits for reviewing the effect the nursing care has had in solving the problem. Such planning may appear too detailed and cumbersome, but its advantage is that every nurse knows exactly what should be done and what the nursing care should achieve, and this makes the extra effort worthwhile.

References

Lelean S. (1974) *Ready for Report, Nurse?* London: RCN
Hunt J. (1979) A comparative study to determine the most effective method of communicating nursing instructions. Final report. The London Hospital. Unpublished report
Salmon (1966) *Report of the Committee on Senior Nursing Staff Structure.* London: HMSO

Chapter 6

Implementation

We hope it is fairly obvious by now that the stages in planning care are not really independant of one another: each stage overlaps the next. This is especially true when discussing nursing instructions which come into both the planning and implementation phases. In the former they are written in the Care Plan, in the latter they are carried out. If the implementation of nursing instructions is to be successful the following points should be thought about carefully:

> how the instructions are to be communicated
> when to carry out the different instructions
> co-ordinating all aspects of care
> actually giving the care
> responsibility and accountability in nursing care

How are instructions communicated?

If patients are to receive the care they require, instructions must be passed on correctly from nurse to nurse. Successful communication (Chapter 5) can be achieved by (*a*) making the instructions specific enough to ensure that no matter who gives the care (or follows the instructions) the interpretation of the instructions will be the same, and (*b*) giving the instructions *in writing* as well as verbally. This combination of specific and written instructions is the ideal. Using a care plan ensures that the instructions are written, and by using a problem-orientated Care Plan each instruction is related to its specific patient nursing problem.

Different wards and units develop their own formats for a Care Plan to suit their own needs. Within a hospital or district, however, some standardisation will be necessary to facilitate the transfer of patients and the use of the Care Plans by the nurses. Whatever the format, the Care Plan becomes the major tool for communicating instructions, and provides a permanent record of these instructions to which all nurses can refer. The Care Plan contains all the information necessary for nursing care: thus it saves time and effort in ward handover reports because it maximises the *useful* information, and reduces the amount of *useless* information, relayed from one nurse to the next.

Communicating instructions successfully

For instructions to be communicated successfully, the following criteria are suggested:

> the instructions should follow a logical step-by-step approach by relating nursing instructions to the patient problems which they are trying to meet;

> the Care Plan format should allow enough room for the nursing instructions to include all the necessary information;

> day-to-day progress notes should be written on a separate part of the Nursing Care Plan but also in close proximity to the nursing instructions so that the progress notes can be written on a problem-solving basis; each problem should be reported on separately;

> the format should allow for the addition of continuation sheets; and all nurses should be able to see at a glance both the short- and the long-range plans for patient care.

"But it will take too much time!"

Although it is necessary to spend some time on writing the initial Care Plan, time is saved in the long run by reducing the amount of information recorded elsewhere, decreasing or eliminating repetition and removing misunderstanding and confusion. Keeping the Care Plan up to date does not take a great deal of time because changes are made only when instructions change: if there is no change in nursing instructions that day, there will be no change in the Care Plan. Progress notes have more meaning and are less repetitive because only the active problems are reported on and all the meaningless phrases traditionally found in present Kardex systems are left out. Instructions like 'four-hourly turns' which are often repeated day after day in the Kardex need not be included in the progress notes because they are permanently written in the Care Plan.

Communicating the Care Plan successfully

The use of a written Care Plan improves verbal communications because handover reporting has greater meaning. Facts and progress are reported on rather than vague generalisations. A common Kardex notation in the traditional system might go something like this: "Mrs. Jones had a good day. Up and about. Specimen or urine N.A.D." This entry really tells nothing about the actual progress Mrs. Jones is making, why her urine is being tested, and what her individual nursing problems are or what the goals for her care might be. A Care Plan with problem-centred progress notes enables reporting to relate to what is actually happening to the patient regarding the progress of each of her problems and towards what goals each nurse must strive. Many nurses, especially junior learners, do not fully understand why they are carrying out many aspects of nursing care. They are just told that Mrs. Jones needs something done but not why it is needed. Problem-centred Care Plans and progress notes provide a system of prescribing nursing care which records the why of nursing care and allows experienced nurses to share their vast wealth of knowledge and skill with learners and the inexperienced.

Problem-centred Care Plans lend themselves to other forms of verbal communication such as nursing rounds and nursing care conferences. A nursing round involves sister or staff nurse using, for example, the afternoon handover time to go with the learners to each patient in the ward. Progress can be reported upon at this time and future care planned. The patient can participate in his care planning, and the round provides a good opportunity for him to ask questions and be given any necessary information and explanations. Obviously, there will at some time be information which may need to be discussed by the nursing staff out of the hearing of the patient (such as with the patient who for some reason has not been told his diagnosis) but aside from this, progress and planning can be discussed on a nursing ward round.

A nursing care conference is a time set aside by the ward nurses to discuss in depth the care, treatment, planning and progress of one patient. It provides a good opportunity for progress to be monitored and for the nursing care to be evaluated to see if goals have been met, and is also an opportune moment to discuss alternative methods of giving nursing care if one particular technique is not working as expected. Priorities in the care for that patient can also be discussed as well as future planning and nursing management. Other health care professionals can come to a nursing care conference and offer suggestions regarding the care of that patient, and this also improves communication within the whole health care team.

What to use at the bedside?

The problem list, goals list and instructions are generally kept, with the progress notes and the initial nursing history, at a central point in the ward (although these can be kept at the bedside). However, some nurses feel the need to have something at each bedside to which they can refer for the basic nursing needs of the patient for that span of duty. Nursing work cards or instruction cards are just that — pre-printed cards which cover all possible aspects of nursing care, filled-in or updated at the beginning of each span of duty or at the time of handover report. Pencil is used so that any changes in the instructions can readily be made (see Fig. 5, Chapter 1). Such work cards are a useful tool, but it must be stressed that they are NOT Care Plans because:

> instructions are erased and changed so there is no permanent record of nursing care;
> forward planning cannot be carried out on work cards because they are only a shift-to-shift indication of what the patient needs;
> retrospective evaluation of nursing care is not possible because the instructions are erased;
> work cards do not list the patients' problems and goals so the rationale for the care is not recorded; and
> priorities cannot be established.

Work cards can, however, be used effectively in conjunction with a problem-orientated Care Plan provided nurses remember that the information is a bedside duplication of what is written in the permanent problem-orientated Care Plan. It is important to note that neither sister nor staff nurse need to, and indeed should not, fill in the work cards — it should be the nurses themselves. If the nurses are allocated their patients before the time of ward handover they will have the relevant work cards in front of them at the time of report and can then make any necessary changes and erasures.

Who updates the Care Plan?

The updating of the permanent problem list, goals list and nursing instructions is left to the ward sister's discretion. She may choose to do this herself or else she can delegate it to her staff nurses or learners if she feels they are capable. This is one aspect of the use of Care Plans which must be left to the individual ward sister to decide.

How to co-ordinate care

In implementing a Care Plan, the nursing care needed by one patient needs to be co-ordinated with other factors such as tests and investigations being carried out on that day on that patient, treatment being given to that patient by other health care professionals, doctors' rounds, the needs of the other patients, and the number of nurses on duty. As the emphasis is on making care individual to the patient this will mean that traditional ward routines need to be re-examined.

Traditionally, nurses try to get all 'the work' (that is, all baths, dressings, bed-making, etc.) completed by noon. If nursing care is to be matched to the individual needs of patients this traditional ward routine must be abandoned. For example, if Mrs. Jones is to have an X-ray examination at 10 a.m. she can be asked whether she wants to have a bath before or after her X-ray. If she chooses to have it afterwards the nurses will plan to bath her in the afternoon. The same is true for other aspects of care. If the same Mrs. Jones has to drink three litres of fluid in 24 hours the nurses must take the X-ray appointment into account. It is ludicrous to plan that 1500 ml of that total be given by her morning nurse, since Mrs. Jones will be in the X-ray department for most of the morning. Instead the afternoon nurse must make a special effort to get Mrs. Jones to drink a lot during the afternoon and evening.

Priorities, of nurse or patient, can be discussed during the handover report. If work cards are being used such priorities can then be indicated in some way, as also can patients' own preferences.

Other health care professionals should have access to the patient's Care Plan so that they, too, may have an overall idea of the patient's total needs. The Care Plan then co-ordinates the patient's nursing needs with the treatment being given by physiotherapists, occupational therapists, etc. With improved communication with these other professionals, the co-ordination between nursing and other care will be improved.

Giving the care

The concepts of task allocation, team nursing and patient allocation have already been discussed in detail (Chapter 2). Individualised care planning requires that a patient-allocation system be used: this ensures continuity of care. The nurse responsible decides when each aspect of care is to be given to her patients and how to go about giving that care. It does not mean that she must work alone and that no one can help her carry out care. On the contrary, there will be aspects of care which are best performed by two nurses, such as bed-making and lifting and turning patients.

Who is responsible?

In patient allocation one nurse is *responsible* and accountable for a group of patients. She decides when and how to carry out care and whether or not she needs another nurse to help her. It also means that the other nurses, sister and the medical staff know who to ask about the care of those patients. It also means that the nurse is accountable should any care not be given to the patient. Most important of all, a patient knows that one nurse is *his* nurse and that he can go to her for information or advice.

The ward sister is ultimately responsible for the nursing care carried out in her ward or department. But in the National Health Service today, over 60% of direct nursing care is carried out by untrained personnel, that is, by learners and auxiliaries. Written Care Plans mean that a sister can be certain that her knowledge and experience are available even when she is not there, and the nursing staff are certain that they are providing care planned by the clinical expert.

It must be remembered that nurses have certain legal responsibilities relating to nursing records. At present, patients' progress is inadequately recorded in many Kardex systems; written Care Plans will help to remedy this deficiency.

To whom are nurses accountable?

Nurses must be accountable to sister or the nurse in charge.

Nursing involves more than just following medical orders. So much of the care a patient receives is based upon nursing decisions. By assuming accountability for the care she gives, a nurse says that her care is professional and that she is giving care which an untrained person cannot give or give as well. Just as medical staff are accountable for the treatment they prescribe and give, so nurses are equally accountable, to their seniors and to their patients, for the nursing care they prescribe and give. Written Care Plans provide the evidence to back up this claim.

A nurse must also be accountable to herself. If she has a reasoned approach to her nursing care and can give sound reasons for her nursing actions, she is approaching her work professionally and scientifically. By documenting her care in a permanent record, the nurse also shares her knowledge and experiences with others, which can be important for the future nursing care of another patient and the extension of knowledge about nursing.

Summary

The implementation stage of care planning is not just carrying out the nursing instructions. Consideration must be given to who gives the instructions, how they are given and, also, to how the implementation of the instructions is recorded. Furthermore, nursing staff have to define their areas of competence and expertise, and accept that they are responsible and accountable for the care they prescribe and give within those areas. Written records that include both a Care Plan and progress notes are therefore, essential tools, for implementation.

Chapter 7

Evaluation

Evaluation is the last phase of nursing care planning. It is essential for determining if the care has been effective, and this involves deciding and measuring how far the specific nursing goals have been met. It is a continuing process that assesses and measures the quality, suitability and degree of success of both the planned nursing care and that care which is actually given — it is, therefore, both an end and a beginning.

The three components of evaluation

In evaluation three components can be studied: structure, process and outcome. *Structure* includes factors like the number and grade of nurses on duty, the type of ward, the nursing workload and the degree of patient dependency. *Process* includes factors such as the content of the plan and the nursing care given or recorded as having been given. *Outcome* includes the results of care in terms either of identifiable changes in the patient's condition directly attributable to the nursing care, or in terms of comparing the expected outcome (the goal) with the actual outcome.

All three components can be studied, firstly, to evaluate the care given to a particular patient and, secondly, to evaluate the Care Plan itself.

The functions of evaluation

As the last phase of the nursing process, evaluation has three major functions:

> to determine whether the goals have been met;
> to provide the information for reassessment of the patient's needs; and
> to discover which nursing actions are most consistently effective in solving a particular nursing problem.

1 Have the nursing goals been met?   It is not easy to measure the effectiveness of nursing care. This can be done, however, for an individual patient by examining whether the nursing goals for that patient have been achieved. For this to be possible the goals have to be stated in quantifiable terms (ie. so that they can be measured) and be realistic. To be measurable, each goal must be written either as a behavioural response of the patient, a verbal response, a specific observation or assessment by the nurse or as a physiological measurement (Fig. 16).

The time or date when any nursing action is to be evaluated is inserted in the Care Plan for that specific problem as it is written. It may be soon, eg. observing the effect of an analgesic after 30 minutes, or delayed, eg. evaluating the teaching of a mentally sub-normal child to dress himself after one month. The important fact is that the nurse predicts when she expects the goal to be achieved, thereby making evaluation possible.

The evaluation itself is a written statement by the nurse of the patient's response to her nursing care at the stated time, ie. it is a statement of what actually has happened. This outcome statement can be included on the Care Plan (Fig. 19). Having the outcome statement on the Care Plan is advantageous. It gives the Care Plan a completeness which makes it useful for easy reference. If outcomes are written only in the progress record they have to be abstracted and this is very time-consuming.

The outcome statement is then compared with the nurse's prediction ie. the goal, and this comparison will show whether or not the goal has been met. In the example shown (Fig. 19) the goals have been met, the pressure sore decreased with time and had 'just healed' by the final review date. A new problem would then be identified either as 'possible recurrence of pressure sore' or 'maintenance of skin integrity', and appropriate goals would again be set and care prescribed. If the goal had not been met by the review date, the prescribed care would need then to have been looked at and perhaps altered and a new review date set. This comparison between goal and outcome shows whether or not the nursing care has been effective, provided the goal was realistic and the care appropriate. By studying the relationship of outcomes to goals during and after the patient's stay in hospital, the nurse can identify those behavioural and physiological changes which have occurred as a result of nursing action. This illuminates progress, or lack of it, towards the desired goals. In

CARE PLAN					

DISCHARGE GOALS

DISCHARGE PLANNING

Tick those needed   Dat

Social services

Community nursing

TTA's and teaching

Out-patients' appt.

Transport

Other

DATE	NO	PATIENT'S NURSING NEEDS/PROBLEMS AND CAUSES OF PROBLEMS (N B Physiological, Psychological, Social and Family problems)	
14·3·80	1	Pressure sore 3 × 2 cm. on sacrum due to lack of mobility.	1 Sore sl in 2 days & a fu smaller
			2 No pre

Fig. 19   Care Plan: showing the outcome statement

this way the nurse obtains the feedback she needs to learn which nursing action was most effective for that particular patient, thereby reducing the need to rely on ritualised patterns of care or on trial and error.

2 Reassessing the patient's needs   A Care Plan is only useful and successful if it is up to date. Frequent revision will be necessary in the case of the acutely ill patient whose condition changes rapidly but, although it should be looked at frequently and changes considered, the Care Plan of a long-term patient may require comparatively little modification.

The reasons for changing a Care Plan are as follows:

a goal has been met and the patient's nursing problem is solved

a goal has not been reached

a new problem has been identified or an existing problem has been alleviated

ordered	OUTCOMES/RESULTS OF NURSING CARE
	1. Pressure sore on sacrum healed by 24.3.80 but skin surface still very fragile. See Problem 8.

GOALS	NURSING INSTRUCTIONS	REVIEW ON/BY	DATE RESOLVED
ould be smaller by 1 cm.		16·3·80	16·3·80
ther 1 cm. in 4 days.		18·3·80	18·3·80
ssure sore.		24·3·80	24·3·80

the goals have been shown to be unrealistic.

When problems are solved or changed they are not erased from the Care Plan. This retention of the original list of problems, plus all the other related information, is essential material for effective evaluation and makes the Care Plan into a valuable permanent record with tremendous potential for research, audit, quality monitoring and teaching material. However, some way of indicating that a problem has been solved or changed is needed. One method is to draw a line through the entry (Fig. 20) in the

PATIENT'S NURSING PROBLEMS

Date noted	Nursing Problems	Date Resolved
14.3.80	Dehydration due to inadequate fluid intake	16.3.80

Fig. 20 Care Plan: indicating that a nursing problem has been solved

same way that a line is drawn through a discontinued drug on some patients' prescription sheets. Another method is to include a 'Data Resolved' column which can then be linked by an arrow to the appropriate problem.

Evaluation of the care given to every patient will ensure that each will receive the best care possible. From the nurse's point of view she needs constantly to think about the care that she is giving and ask herself the following questions:

> Do I have all the information I need?
> Have I got my priorities right?
> Are my goals realistic?
> Have I helped the patient to understand the goals?
> Are the nursing instructions being implemented as written on the Care Plan?
> Were the instructions the right ones for reaching the goals?
> Has the nursing care brought about a positive change in the patient's condition?
> Have all changes in condition and all information been fully documented?
> Does everyone understand, and give the same interpretation to, what I have written?

The evaluation of care, recorded as the actual outcome, does not provide for a very detailed daily record, or for recording information which may be of very temporary importance or for recording the intermediate stages towards the solution of a problem. A progress record fulfils these functions (Fig. 4). It can be written by the nurses during each span of duty; *during* is, perhaps, the word which needs particular emphasis, since the progress record should be a continuing account of the patient's day and not an end-of-shift report. The progress record is best written in terms of individual problems and how the problems are being resolved or alleviated, but the narrative method now commonly used by nurses can be retained.

3 Matching nursing plans and actions Evaluation can also be used to record the effectiveness of nursing care in solving the nursing problems of a specific patient. This is of particular importance in two ways: firstly, when a problem has been particularly difficult to solve and has required several approaches before the right one has been identified; and secondly, when a patient has to be re-admitted either for regular treatment (eg. cytotoxic therapy), because of a deterioration in an existing condition (eg. chronic bronchitis), or for a new illness or accident. In all such instances the knowledge gained during previous admissions on the most effective way of dealing with that patient's nursing problems not only saves time, but also demonstrates to the patient that the nurses understand his particular needs.

Evaluation of the Care Plan

Evaluation has a wider application than simply assessing the effectiveness of the nursing care given to a particular patient, vital though this aspect is. It can also be used to evaluate the Care Plans themselves, the competence of the nurses' planning and giving of care, and the overall standard of performance.

A Care Plan has to show evidence of a satisfactory level of knowledge and expertise. It can, therefore, be evaluated by 'experts' to determine whether it is of a satisfactory standard. Such an evaluation can be done on the basis of each patient's care, or by comparing a Care Plan with pre-specified criteria involving many previous patients. Evaluation of the Care Plan is essential because the care given reflects the standard of the care prescribed; if the latter is low then its is likely that the care the patient receives will be low. Clearly, if the nurse who prescribes by writing the Care Plan is also the nurse who gives the care, it is much easier to identify this relationship.

Evaluation of the Care Plan must cover all aspects of the plan; whether the patient's nursing problems accurately reflect the patient's needs; whether the goals are correct, and, equally important, whether they are realistic; whether the nursing actions are the most appropriate for meeting the goals and can be carried out within the resources available, and whether the time allowed before evaluating the results of the care is appropriate and realistic. The two examples overleaf demonstrate adequate and inadequate planning in relation to a similar problem.

Evaluating nurses' knowledge

The writing of nursing Care Plans is a very useful means of assessing a nurse's knowledge, and how well she can apply knowledge and use her ability to interpret information. Identifying nursing problems from the available data, setting goals which are

ADEQUATE PLANNING

Problem	Goal	Instructions	Review on/by
Chest pain caused by myocardial infarction	No chest pain	1 Give analgesics every 4 hours as prescribed 2 Give glyceryl trinitrate as required 3 Ask patient whether he has pain 4 Report to sister if patient remains in pain	$\frac{1}{2}$ hour & $3\frac{1}{2}$ hours after analgesia

INADEQUATE PLANNING

Problem	Goal	Instructions	Review on/by
Chest pain caused by myocardial infarction	No chest pain	Give analgesics if patient asks for them	4-hourly or drug rounds

realistic and detailing the nursing care necessary to achieve these goals, are the criteria which provide ward sisters, nurse managers and tutors with a very informative and accurate assessment of a nurse's knowledge and competence. The completion of the progress notes and of the outcome statements and the use the nurse makes of this continuing information not only augment the sister's or tutor's assessment of her knowledge, but also demonstrate the nurse's ability to translate the nursing instructions into practice.

Evaluating standards of care

Finally, to revert to a point mentioned at the beginning of this chapter, evaluation of Care Plans can be used to assess the standard of care. Nurses often complain that the standard of care is steadily declining, but the fact is that they have no precise means of measuring acceptable standards and therefore cannot make such a judgement. One of the main reasons for this is the lack of detailed and accurate records of the care planned for, and given to, the patient. The development and use of Care Plans will make it possible for individual nurses, groups of nurses, ward sisters, nurse managers, teaching staff and researchers to look at what is happening, monitor the nursing care that patients receive, compare the care given on different wards and evaluate different approaches to the same nursing problem. All will, for the first time, be able to obtain data never before available about the day-to-day practice of nursing, which opens up tremendous opportunities for nurses to examine and research clinical nursing practice.

Summary

Evaluation may be the last phase in care planning but it is as essential as all the other phases. Evaluation as described in this chapter is new to nurses, but if we are to develop *nursing,* then evaluation must become an accepted part of every nurse's practice. Care Plans will ensure the information is recorded. The evaluation of critical examination of that information will ensure that high standards of care are set and maintained.

Helpful Hints

What are Nursing Care Plans?

Nursing Care Plans are written for individual patients and are a practical way of putting the nursing process to work. They are not the same thing as the nursing process, although there is a definite relationship between the activity of producing Nursing Care Plans and the philosophy of the nursing process. Producing a Nursing Care Plan involves assessing the patient's needs and planning appropriate care. The nursing care can then be given, or modified and adapted as necessary, using the written record called the Nursing Care Plan; furthermore, care given can subsequently be evaluated. A Nursing Care Plan is, therefore, a practical tool which helps nurses to give individualised care to patients.

A Nursing Care Plan has four purposes. It provides an assessment of the patient's needs; details of the planned care; a description of how this was implemented, and an evaluation of the outcomes for the patient. These steps correspond to the four stages of the nursing process. Learning about Nursing Care Plans, and gaining practice in their use, should help nurses towards a clearer understanding of the principles of the nursing process.

It is important that readers should understand the terminology which has been used throughout the book, to avoid the danger of confusion. When we talk about *Nursing Care Plans,* (ie. capital initial letters and preceded by Nursing) we mean all the paperwork which is needed to put the nursing process to work, including the patient's history, his progress notes, and the planned programme of patient care itself.

However, when we speak of the whole process of decision-making and recording which is necessary in order to produce a Nursing Care Plan, we have termed this activity *care planning* (ie. without 'nursing' and without capital initials). On occasion, particularly in Chapters 3 and 5, we will need to refer to that part of the whole Nursing Care Plan which contains just the written list of the patient's problems, and corresponding actions and goals. We have called this document the *Care Plan,* but wherever we have used this phrase we have differentiated it from the whole Nursing Care Plan.

In the United Kingdom there is an increasing interest in and emphasis on making nursing care more individual, as well as planning it on a more scientific basis. We believe this to be necessary, and that it will have important benefits for the patient; we have therefore set out some hints for nurses, nurse administrators and nurse tutors who are interested in implementing Care Plans or the nursing process which may be useful before embarking on large or even small-scale implementation of the approaches we have described.

1 Find some people who are already implementing Nursing Care Plans or some form of individualised care planning and talk to them. Ask them to come and speak to others in your hospital.
2 Start small. Do not attempt to create a Nursing Care Plan package to try on a ward and then expect the ward to begin implementation straight away.
3 Try one thing at a time — start with, for example, patient allocation or using individual work cards or perhaps nursing histories.
4 Find one ward sister who is at least interested in trying to use Nursing Care Plans.
5 Make sure the new system is practicable under existing staffing levels and workload.
6 Go slowly. Do not rush people or force them into accepting a completely new system straight away.
7 Involve the School of Nursing as soon as possible to provide both ward and school-based teaching.
8 Organise workshops or in-service courses for qualified nurses to teach them the techniques of implementation.
9 Listen to, and incorporate suggestions from wards which are using Nursing Care Plans.
10 Give the nurses as much praise and encouragement as is justified. Concentrate on the patients and nurse and not on the system alone.

Care planning using patient-centred Nursing Care Plans based on the nursing process has a number of advantages over other methods of planning and recording nursing care:

1 When presented and taught step-by-step it is easy to understand and more likely to be adopted at ward level.
2 Nurses at all levels of training and seniority begin to think of the reason/s behind the prescribed care, so that care is not given just because 'Sister says so' or because 'that's the way

we've always done it', but because it is known to be effective.

3 Setting goals ensures that nurses and patients know what they are trying to achieve, and allows the care to be evaluated in terms of whether or not the goals have been met.

4 It lends itself to a completely new method of teaching learners.

5 It creates further possibilities for multi-disciplinary approaches to care by its easy accessibility to doctors, physiotherapists and other members of the health care team. It is possible to use this type of format as a basis for a problem-orientated patient record which includes all problems, goals and actions (medical, nursing, etc.) defined by all members of the health care team.

6 It encourages learners to take a more active part in planning patient care under guidance from senior members of staff. This involvement will make nursing more stimulating and challenging to learners.

7 It encourages patients to take part in the planning of their care, by enabling them to know the goals towards which they can aspire, and gives them something positive to work towards.

8 Nursing becomes more effective in that care does not continue to be used if it is not proving to be effective. This means that the patient will not be given nursing care which is not working.

The nursing process has been talked and written about at some length. Ultimately, however, the only test of the validity of the approaches described in this book lies in their implementation and the effect that this will have on nurses and the well-being of patients. Care Plans using a problem-orientated approach are tangible evidence of the implementation of the nursing process. They are exciting and challenging to use. They are the nursing process at work.

Section IV

A Look at the Literature

Chapter 8 A Reading Guide
Chapter 9 Bibliography

This section provides more detailed information about the theory of care planning and the nursing process. Chapter 8 is a reading guide to those texts that we have found most helpful, and Chapter 9 an extensive bibliography for those who wish to pursue their study of care planning and the nursing process.

Chapter 8

A Reading Guide

Introduction

An enormous amount of material has been published on all aspects of planning nursing care under such headings as the nursing process, total patient care and patient allocation. Some of the literature is theoretical in content, while some is more practical; some has been written for nurses with a good background knowledge and understanding of care planning and its components, and some for nurses with very little. A comprehensive literature review in this book would be very long and cumbersome and of limited value to nurses who wish to learn about the practical application of care planning, and is not intended here. The books and articles recommended in this chapter are a subjective and necessarily arbitrary choice, and consist largely of readings that have proved helpful and which the authors have recommended to nursing colleagues.

The material in this chapter is in three sections at different levels of understanding of care planning. The first section will be particularly useful to those nurses with little related background knowledge and who are more interested in implementing Nursing Care Plans than in the theoretical background. Once they have reached a basic level of understanding, however, it is hoped that they will wish to progress to the other sections of this reading guide. The second section is designed for nurses who have a fairly sound basic understanding of care planning, whether they themselves have implemented care plans or not, and who would like a guide to more advanced information. The literature referred to in these first two sections covers the four stages of care planning — assessment, planning, implementation and evaluation — and includes all the theory needed for practical purposes in most wards and departments. The third and final section briefly looks at some of the theories behind the planning of care and the nursing process. The titles of all the books and journals mentioned in each section are listed both at the end of the chapter and in the comprehensive bibliography which forms the next chapter and, therefore, only the author's name and date of publication are given in the text.

Basic reading

The first book which we would recommend to nurses with a limited amount of background knowledge about care planning and the nursing process is a small, 60-page volume by Rehman (1976). The author concentrates on the practical implementation of care plans and avoids delving into theoretical matters. Good, basic, practical guidance is given about each of the four stages of the nursing process and the book is written and set out in a very readable way. The author does further sub-divide the four stages of care planning, which can be confusing to the beginner.

Several useful articles have appeared in British and American nursing journals. Duberley (1977), in a short but easy-to-understand article, discusses the changes in thinking which are needed to make care planning a reality. Lewis (1968) has also written on the same topic. Two equally practical articles on the implementation of Nursing Care Plans by Little & Carnevalli (1967; 1971) are also worth looking at.

The easiest way to implement Nursing Care Plans is to begin by using a nursing admission history. Even with no knowledge of the theoretical background and no wish to be involved further in Nursing Care Plans, the nursing history is a useful and practical tool used to gather information about a patient and at the same time to make the patient feel that he is of interest and importance to the nursing staff. Taking a history also helps to establish a good nurse-patient relationship. Many articles have been written which can provide useful, practical information on how to develop and use nursing histories and what to do with the information which has been gained from them. Two such articles are those by McCain (1965), who outlines the practical aspects of making a nursing assessment of a patient through taking an admission history, and by McPheteridge (1968) who discusses how the application of the important information obtained by taking a nursing history well makes the subsequent nursing care very individual to that patient.

Another approach to care planning which is being made by nurses in the UK is to change from task allocation to patient allocation. Nurses who are interested in learning how other professional colleagues have implemented patient allocation should read Matthews' articles (1975), which are relevant to British nursing and can be helpful for any nurse who seeks practical advice on how to change from task-orientated care to patient-orientated care. Pembrey's article (1975) on changing from task assignment is also recommended. It deals with the adjustments needed in the management style of the ward sister in order to implement patient allocation.

Further reading

In this section we hope to provide some guidance for nurses who intend or have begun to use Nursing Care Plans, and the books and articles mentioned are aimed at those who have a sound basic understanding of Nursing Care Plans. While some of the texts recommended contain chapters on theory, most of their content is about the practice of care planning. Probably the best text at this level is that by Mayers (1972), providing a wealth of information to those nurses who are already familiar with the basic concept. Mayers presents a systematic method of collecting and organising patient information so that care is planned and given in a more personalised way than in the traditional manner. She discusses the problem-solving approach to care planning where nurses use the information obtained from a nursing history to identify problems, set goals or objectives and decide what nursing care will meet the goals to solve the patient's problems. Mayers has nursed both in hospital and in the community, as well as being a nurse educator, and her book explores in all these three areas how the problem-solving approach can be implemented, and the problems that are faced by nurses when trying to implement this type of individualised care. She gives examples of several different nursing history formats and good practical guidance on defining patients' nursing problems and setting goals.

Nurses who have read about the nursing process will be aware that the one aspect of the four components of care planning which is hardly ever carried out at present is evaluation. Mayers devotes an entire chapter to the concept of evaluating nursing care by first deciding what it is hoped to achieve and then looking back to see if it has been achieved. However, this book is American and in consequence American terms and phrases are used which may be unfamiliar to British nurses; even so, it is one of the most useful books on the subject of planning care.

Yura & Walsh (1973) also present a practical approach to care planning for those who have some background understanding of the nursing process. This also is an American book but it gives helpful information on the different components of the process of planning care. However, the book does discuss in great depth the theoretical approaches to nursing. These authors also include a comprehensive historical account of the development of the nursing process over the past few decades, which shows how the process began as an educational idea and became a practical reality in the planning and giving of nursing care. This chapter also provides a good basic description of many nursing theories and is a good introduction to this topic.

Marriner (1975) has written a book for those nurses who wish to further their understanding of planning nursing care. She discusses the four stages of care planning in great depth and includes selected readings from journals to illustrate her points. The assessment chapter is particularly recommended since it discusses interviewing techniques and how to use both the patient's verbal and non-verbal responses in making a nursing assessment and stresses the importance of listening to all that the patient is saying.

The last book to be included in this section is by Little & Carnevalli (1969). Again, the main value is its problem-solving approach and emphasis on evaluating nursing care to see if the set goals have been achieved. These authors also bring out the point that planning nursing care is not just an extra job for nurses but an essential job which must be given its due importance. There is also a good chapter on communication — between nurses, medical staff and patients.

Although a great deal of the literature is American the amount of British work available is increasing; for example, a series of articles on the nursing process was published in the *Nursing Times* during 1977. The introductory article to this series by Kratz is invaluable. She says that the nursing process is simply a 'kind of prescription' of how nurses do or ought to do their work.

She also warns nurses to reject the idea that 'they have always done' the nursing process by pointing out that, traditionally, nurses gave care based on information received from doctors, medical records, what the patient told them while having a bed bath, and what the ward routine dictated. With the nursing process, patient care revolves around a *systematic* recording of information collected by nurses solely for planning nursing care and the implementation of that planned care. Kratz goes on to say that the nursing process is 'new' because of the problem-solving approach and because of the inbuilt evaluation of nursing care. The remaining articles in that particular series were by Crow and illustrate the kind of detailed care planning that can be carried out using a problem-solving approach. Although the care plans in these articles were completed as an educational exercise, what comes across most clearly and does have very practical relevance is that although the two patients whose care studies are presented had the same medical diagnosis, their nursing care was very different because the individual needs to be met and problems to be solved were very different.

Theory

This last section outlines three of the theories which have been used as a basis for the development of care planning, namely:

> general systems theory
> human need theory
> Roy adaptation model

A selection of other theories and models have been and are being used. What is important is not so much which theory is used but that nurses define nursing and plan nursing care within a coherent and clearly stated theoretical framework.

General systems theory   The systems theory is discussed in great detail by Yura & Walsh (1973). They define a system as that which provides the structure through which a whole may be divided into its component parts so that the relationship between these parts can be studied and manipulated. It also provides a structure whereby unconnected parts may be integrated into an organised whole. Any system can be divided into sub-systems, each of which may carry out a purpose, which enables the general purpose of the system to be achieved. Yura & Walsh relate this to nursing by looking at nursing in terms of the 'health care system' as a whole with nursing being one of the sub-systems. The 'health care system' is a system within society, society being the 'supra-system' (see Figs. 21 & 22). Yura & Walsh then go on to explore the interaction and action which takes place between and within the systems to discuss the psychological, physiological and environmental implications and how the nursing process is central in the feedback of information.

Human need theory The human need theory quite simply says that man's motivation is towards meeting his needs. A human need is defined as an internal tension which results in a change of some sort within man's system. Maslow's Hierarchy of Needs (1962) is the most commonly used model for the human need theory. Maslow says that the realization of a person's full potential is affected by the satisfaction (or lack of satisfaction) of his basic needs. He devised a hierarchy of needs at five levels. Fundamental physical needs must be met first and so they comprise the first level, which include the need for air, food, sleep, rest, sex, exercise and activity. Physical needs dominate man: if his basic needs are not met his total human capacity will be directed towards satisfying them. It is only when his needs are met that man can think about meeting other needs which are further up in Maslow's hierarchy.

The second level of needs, according to Maslow, includes the need for uninterrupted routine and safety. Man needs to live in a predictable, orderly world and when it is not, he concentrates his efforts on filling this gap. Once this occurs, he can proceed to the third level which includes the need for loving (which involves both the giving and receiving of love) and belonging. The absence of these is deeply felt. The fourth level is the need for esteem. Once the previous needs are met man needs to have a stable, firmly-based, wholesome evaluation of himself and respect for others. If this need is not met, man feels inferior and tries to overcome these feelings. The last level in the hierarchy is self-actualisation. This means that man needs to feel self-fulfilled. In short, when all other needs are met, man will strive towards feeling that he is doing what he wants to do in life and will grow restless and discontented if this need is not met.

According to Yura & Walsh, the human need theory states that the preservation, the fostering, the maintenance and the meeting of all individual human needs is the territory of nursing,

SOCIETY OR ENVIRONMENT

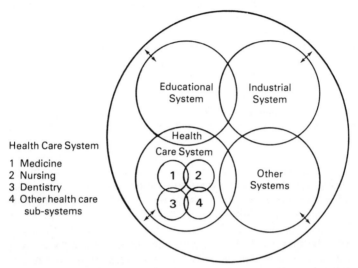

Fig. 21   The supra-system: society or environment. If the circle no. 2 denoting the nursing sub-system is enlarged, it could be represented as in Figure 22

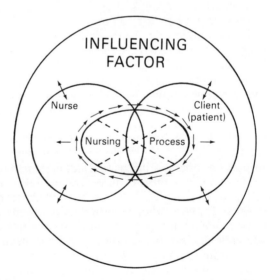

Fig. 22   Sub-system no. 2: Nursing (within the Health Care system)

and this means that nursing must strive to meet patients' needs.

The application of the human need theory to planning nursing care is quite clear. Nursing must meet all human needs, beginning with those on the first level of the hierarchy and continuing upward, and through the identification of unfulfilled needs nursing care must be planned to attempt to satisfy them.

Roy adaptation model Riehl & Roy (1974) explore several models for nursing practice, including the two mentioned above. They also discuss the Roy adaptation model, set out by Sister Callista Roy in the United States. This is the theoretical model used successfully by the Department of Nursing at Manchester University. Very briefly, the Roy adaptation model says that man adapts to illness in four ways — physiologically; in terms of self concept; in his rôle function; and in his dependence. So, when assessing a patient, the assessment must be in terms of these four adaptations. Other articles which explore Roy's theory can be found in *Nursing Outlook* (1970; 1971; 1973; 1975).

Roy says that nurses must gather information and form conclusions (or nursing diagnoses) based upon this information. How the patient adapts to these statements of need forms the basis of the Nursing Care Plan.

This section only outlines briefly three of the theories in current use and is written with the sole objective of providing a starting point for nurses who wish to pursue further study of care planning. The authors believe that the use of these theories will stimulate nurses and ultimately lead not only to the further development of nursing theory but also to the development and improvement of nursing practice.

References

Section 1: Basic Reading

Duberley J. (1977) How will the change strike me and you. *Nursing Times,* **73** (10 Nov.), 1736-38
Lewis L. (1968) This I believe ... about the nursing process. *Nursing Outlook,* **16** (5), 26-29
Little D. & Carnevalli D. (1967) Nursing care plans: let's be practical about them. *Nursing Forum,* No. 1, 61-76

Little D. & Carnevalli D. (1971) The nursing care planning system. *Nursing Outlook,* **19** (3), 164-167

Matthews A. (1975) Patient allocation – a review. *Nursing Times,* **71** (July 10, 17, 24, 31)

McCain R. (1965) Nursing by assessment – not intuition. *American Journal of Nursing,* April, 82-84

McPheteridge M. (1968) Nursing history: one means to personalize care. *American Journal of Nursing,* Jan., 68-75

Pembrey S. (1975) From work routines to patient assignment: an experiment in ward management. *Nursing Times,* **71** (Nov.), 1768-72

Rehman J. (1976) *Writing Patient Care Plans.* San Diego: Professional Lecture Series Inc

Section 2: Further Reading

Crow J. (1977) The nursing process 1, 2 & 3. *Nursing Times,* **73** (June 16, 23, 30)

Kratz C. (1977) The nursing process. *Nursing Times,* **73** (June 9), 854-855

Little D. & Carnevalli D. (1969) *Nursing Care Planning.* Philadelphia: Lippincott

Marriner A. (1975) *The Nursing Process: A Scientific Approach to Nursing Care.* St. Louis: Mosby

Mayers M. (1978) *A Systematic Approach to Nursing Care Plans.* New York: Appleton-Century-Crofts

Yura H. & Walsh M. (1973) *The Nursing Process.* New York: Appleton-Century-Crofts

Section 3: Theory

Maslow A. (1962) *Toward a Psychology of Being.* Princeton, N. J.: Van Nostrand

Riehl J. P. & Roy C. (1974) *Conceptual Models for Nursing Practice.* New York: Appleton-Century-Crofts

Roy C. (1970) Adaptation: a conceptual framework for nursing. *Nursing Outlook,* **18** (3), 42-45

Roy C. (1971) Adaptation: a basis for nursing practice. *Nursing Outlook,* **19** (4), 254-257

Roy C. (1973) Adaptation: implications for curriculum change. *Nursing Outlook,* **21** (3), 163-168

Roy C. (1975) A diagnostic classification system for nursing. *Nursing Outlook,* **23** (2), 90-94

Chapter 9

Bibliography

The following is a fairly comprehensive bibliography on the nursing process, individualised Nursing Care Plans and related topics. The sources quoted are grouped by subject, as indicated below, with book and journal articles listed separately:

> The Nursing Process — General
>
> Admission Histories, Patient Assessment and Nursing
>> Diagnoses
>
> Nursing Care Plans and Problem-Orientated Records
>
> Primary Nursing and Total Patient Care
>
> Patient-Centred Care
>
> Patient Allocation
>
> Team Nursing.

The nursing process — general

BOOKS

Kratz C. (ed) (1979) *The Nursing Process.* London: Baillière Tindall

Marriner A. (1975) *The Nursing Process: A Scientific Approach to Nursing Care.* St. Louis: Mosby

Orlando I. J. (1972) *The Discipline and Teaching of Nursing Process: An Evaluative Study.* New York: Putnam

Riehl J. P. & Roy C. (1974) *Conceptual Models for Nursing Practice.* New York: Appleton-Century-Crofts

Sundeen S. J. *et al.* (1976) *Nurse-Client Interaction: Implementing the Nursing Process.* St Louis: Mosby

Travelbee J. (1969) *Intervention in Psychiatric Nursing Process in 1:1 Relationship.* Philadelphia: F. A. Davis

University of Kansas Medical Center Department of Nursing
    Education (1974) *Case Studies of Nursing Intervention.*
    New York: McGraw-Hill
Yura H. & Walsh M. B. (1978) *The Nursing Process: Assessing,
    Planning, Implementing, Evaluating.* New York:
    Appleton-Century-Crofts

JOURNAL ARTICLES

Bergeron H. J. & Zagornik A. (1968) Teaching nursing process
    to beginning students. *Nursing Outlook,* **16** (7), 32-38
Bomar P. J. (1975) The nursing process in the care of a hostile
    pregnant adolescent. *Maternal-Child Nursing Journal,* **4**
    (2), 95-100
Carlson S. (1972) A practical approach to the nursing process.
    American Journal of Nursing, **72** (9), 1589-91
Crow J. (1977) The nursing process—1: theoretical background.
    Nursing Times, **73** (June 16), 892-896
Crow J. (1977) The nursing process—2: how and why to take a
    nursing history. *Nursing Times,* **73** (June 23), 950-957
Crow J. (1977) The nursing process—3: a nursing history ques-
    tionnaire for two patients. *Nursing Times,* **73** (June 30),
    978-982 (see also pp. 983-994 for Care Studies and centre
    pages for Care Plans)
Daubenmire M. J. & King I. M. (1973) Nursing process models:
    a systems approach. *Nursing Outlook,* **21** (8), 512-517
Duberley J. (1977) How will the change strike me and and you.
    Nursing Times, **73** (Nov. 10), 1736-38
Goodwin J. O. & Edwards B. S. (1975) Developing a computer
    program to assist the nursing process: phase 1 — from
    systems analysis to an expendable program. *Nursing
    Research,* **4** (July-Aug.), 229-305
Griffiths E. W. (1971) Nursing process: a patient with respira-
    tory dysfunction. *Nursing Clinics of North America,* **6** (3),
    141-154
Hargreaves I. (1975) The nursing process: the key to individual-
    ised care. *Nursing Times,* **71** (Aug. 28), occasional papers
    89-92
Hegyvary S. T. & Haussman R. K. D. (1976) The relationship of
    nursing process and patient outcomes. *Journal of Nursing
    Administration,* **6** (9), 18-21

Jones C. (1977) The nursing process: individualised care. *Nursing Mirror,* **144** (Oct. 13), 13-14

Lewis L. (1968) This I believe . . . about the nursing process. *Nursing Outlook,* **16** (5), 26-29

Kratz C. (1977) The nursing process. *Nursing Times,* **73** (June 9), 854-855

McClure E. & Warwick J. (1977) The nursing process studied in Toronto. *Nursing Mirror,* **144** (Feb. 10), 55-57

MacFarlane J. (1975) What do we mean by care? *Nursing Mirror,* **141** (Oct. 2), 47-48

MacFarlane J. (1976) A charter for caring. *Journal of Advanced Nursing,* **1** (1), 187-196

Nursing Times (1977) The nursing process (W H O Regional Office for Europe meeting at Nottingham to examine aspects of the nursing process). *Nursing Times,* **73** (Jan. 6), 11

R C N Association of Nursing Education — Wessex Region (1977) Introducing the nursing process. *Nursing Times,* **73** (May 26), 763

Rubel M. (1976) Coming to grips with the nursing process. *Supervisor Nurse,* **7** (2), 30-32, 34, 36, 38-39

Schaefer J. (1974) The inter-relatedness of decision making and the nursing process. *American Journal of Nursing,* **71** (10), 1852-55

Scottish National Nursing & Midwifery Consultative Committee (1976) The process of nursing. *Nursing Mirror,* **143** (July 1), 55-57

Winslow S. S. (1977) Pain: part 2. A personalised approach (using the nursing process to determine patients' needs). *Journal of Practical Nursing,* **27** (2), 16-17, 34, 41

Admission histories, patient assessment and nursing diagnoses

BOOKS

Fowkes W. C. & Hunn V. K. (1974) *Clinical Assessment for the Nurse-Practitioner.* St Louis: Mosby

Gebbie K. & Lavin M. (1975) *Classification of Nursing Diagnoses.* St Louis: Mosby

Hobson L. B. (1975) *Examination of the Patient: A Text for Nursing and Allied Health Personnel.* New York: McGraw-Hill

Sana J. M. & Judge R. D. (Eds) (1975) *Physical Appraisal Methods in Nursing Practice.* Boston: Little, Brown

Seedor M. M. (1974) *The Physical Assessment: a Programmed Unit of Study for Nurses.* New York: Teachers' College Press

JOURNAL ARTICLES

American Journal of Nursing (1974) Patient assessment: taking a patient's history — programmed instruction. *American Journal of Nursing,* **74** (2), 293-324

Aspinall M. J. (1976) Nursing diagnosis — the weak link. *Nursing Outlook,* **24** (7), 433-437

Bircher A. U. (1975) On the development and classification of diagnosis. *Nursing Forum,* **14** (1), 10-29

Brown M. M. (1974) Epidemiological approach to the study of clinical nursing diagnosis. *Nursing Forum,* **13** (4), 346-359

Durand M. & Prince R. (1966) Nursing diagnosis process and decision. *Nursing Forum,* **5** (4), 50-64

Fry J. & Majumdar B. (1974) Basic physical assessment. *Canadian Nurse,* **70** (5) 17-22

Fuller D. & Rosenaur J. A. (1974) A patient assessment guide. *Nursing Outlook,* **22** (7), 460-462

Gordon M. (1976) Nursing diagnoses and the diagnostic process. *American Journal of Nursing,* **76** (8), 1298-1300

Hefferin E. A. & Hunter R. E. (1975) Nursing assessment and care plan statements. *Nursing Research,* **24** (Sept.-Oct), 360-366

Hagopian G. & Kilpack V. (1974) Baccalaureate students learn assessment skills. *Nursing Outlook,* **22** (7), 454-456

Kamorita M. I. (1963) Nursing diagnoses. *American Journal of Nursing,* **63** (12), 83-86

Langner S. R. (1973) The nursing process and the interview. *Occupational Health Nursing,* **21** (12), 19-23

Lynaugh J. E. & Bates B. (1974) Physical diagnosis: a skill for all nurses? *American Journal of Nursing,* **74** (1), 58-59

McCain R. E. (1965) Nursing by assessment — not intuition. *American Journal of Nursing,* **65** (4), 82-84

McPheteridge M. (1968) Nursing history: one means to personalize care. *American Journal of Nursing,* **68** (1), 68-75

Mahomet A. D. (1975) Nursing diagnosis for the O R nurse. *A O R N Journal,* **22** (5), 709-711

Matheny A. (1967) A guide for interviewing. *American Journal of Nursing,* **67** (10), 2088-90

Mundinger M. O. & Jauron G. (1975) Developing a nursing diagnosis. *Nursing Outlook,* **23** (2), 94-98

Murray J. B. (1963) Self knowledge and the nursing interview. *Nursing Forum,* **2** (1), 66-78

Myers N. (1973) Nursing diagnosis. *Nursing Times,* **69** (Sept. 20), 1229-30

Nursing Clinics of North America (1971) Symposium on assessment as part of the nursing process. *Nursing Clinics of North America,* **6** (1), 113-200

Roy C. (1975) The impact of nursing diagnosis. *A O R N Journal,* **21** (6), 1023-30

Smith D. (1964) Myth and method in nursing practice. *American Journal of Nursing,* **64** (2), 68-72

Smith D. (1968) A clinical nursing tool. *American Journal of Nursing,* **68** (11), 2384-88

U S Public Health Service (1959) A study of the effect of different nursing actions. Grant no. G N 62651-A

U S Public Health Service (1963) Interactions of patients and staff on a medical ward. Grant no. G M 10050-1

Wesseling E. (1972) Automating the nursing history and care plan. *Journal of Nursing Administration,* **11** (May-June), 34-38

Nursing care plans and problem-orientated records

BOOKS

American Hospital Association (1966) *Nursing Care Plans.* Chicago: Hospital Research & Educational Trust

Berni R. & Readey H. (1974) *Problem-Oriented Medical Record Implementation.* St Louis: Mosby

Bjorn J. & Cross H. (1970) *Problem-Oriented Practice.* Chicago: Modern Hospital Press

Bower F. L. (1972) *The Process of Planning Nursing Care: A Theoretical Model.* St Louis: Mosby

Eckelberry G. K. (1971) *Administration of Comprehensive Nursing Care: The Nature of Professional Practice.* New York: Appleton-Century-Crofts

Hunt J. M. (1978) The planning of nursing care. In Tiffany R. (Ed) *Oncology for Nurses and Health Care Professionals.* London: Allen & Unwin

Hurst J. & Walker J. (1972) *The Problem-Oriented System*. New York: Medcom

Johnson M. *et al.* (1973) *Problem Solving in Nursing Practice*. Dubuque U.S.A.: Wm. Brown

Kraegal J. M. *et al.* (1974) *Patient Care Systems*. Philadelphia: Lippincott

Larkin P. & Backer B. (1977) *Problem-Oriented Nursing Assessment*. New York: McGraw-Hill

Lewis L. (1970) *Planning Patient Care*. Dubuque USA: Wm. Brown

Little D. E. & Carnevalli D. L. (1969) *Nursing Care Planning*. Philadelphia: Lippincott

McManus R. L. (1952) Assumption of functions of nursing. In *Regional Planning for Nursing and Nursing Education*. Report of Conference, Plymouth, New Hampshire, 1950. New York: Columbia University Teachers' College Bureau of Publications

Mayers M. (1972) *A Systematic Approach to Nursing Care Plans*. New York: Appleton-Century-Crofts

Mayers M. (1974) *Standard Nursing Care Plans*. Palo Alto USA: K/P Co. Medical Systems

Neelon F. & Ellis G. (1974) *A Syllabus of Problem-Oriented Patient Care*. Boston: Little, Brown

Rehman J. (1976) *Writing Patient Care Plans*. San Diego: Professional Lecture Series Inc

Saxton D. F. & Hyland P. (1975) *Planning and Implementing Nursing Intervention*. St Louis: Mosby

Vaughan-Wroebel B. & Henderson B. (1976) *The Problem-Oriented System in Nursing*. St Louis: Mosby

Vitale B. *et al.* (1974) *A Problem Solving Approach to Nursing Care Plans*. St. Louis: Mosby.

Walker J. B. *et al.* (1976) *Dynamics of Problem-Oriented Approaches: Patient Care and Documentation*. Philadelphia: Lippincott

Weed L. (1969) *Medical Records, Medical Education and Patient Care*. Cleveland: Case Western Reserve University

JOURNAL ARTICLES

Baldwin S. M. (1976) Made to measure care. *Nursing Times,* **72** (Mar. 25), 468-469

Christensen J. C. (1975) Planning nursing care. *New Zealand Nursing Journal,* **69** (April), 3-7

Ciuca R. L. (1972) Over the years with the nursing care plan. *Nursing Outlook,* **20** (11), 706-711

Collingwood M. P. (1975) The nursing care plan as a basis for an information system based on individualised patient care. *Nursing Times,* **71** (Mar. 20), 21-22, occasional paper

Copp L. A. (1972) Improved patient care through evaluation — part 3: your plan of nursing care. *Bedside Nurse,* **5** (Sept.), 25-29

Cornell S. A. & Brush F. (1971) Systems approach to nursing care plans. *American Journal of Nursing,* **71** (July), 1376-78

Francis (1967) This thing called problem solving. *Journal of Nursing Education,* **6** (Nov. 19), 27-30

Garant C. (1972) A basis for care. *American Journal of Nursing,* **72** (4), 699-701

Grant N. (1975) The nursing care plan. *Nursing Times,* **71** (Mar. 27), 25-28, occasional papers

Harris B. L. (1970) Who needs written care plans anyway? *American Journal of Nursing,* **70** (10), 2136-38

Heath J. K. & Griffith E. W. (1972) An experience in rôle implementation. *Journal of Nursing Education,* **11** (April), 13-20

Henderson V. (1973) On nursing care plans and their history. *Nursing Outlook,* **21** (6), 378-379

Josten L. V. *et al.* (1972) Staff plan to minimize paper nursing. *American Journal of Nursing,* **72** (3), 492-493

Kelly N. C. (1966) Nursing care plans. *Nursing Outlook,* **14** (5), 61-64

Little D. E. & Carnevalli D. L. (1967) Nursing care plans: let's be practical about them. *Nursing Forum,* **6** (1), 61-76

Little D. E. & Carnevalli D. L. (1971) The nursing care planning system. *Nursing Outlook,* **19** (3), 164-167

McCloskey J. C. (1975) The nursing care plan: past, present and uncertain future. *Nursing Forum,* **14**, 364-382

McCloskey J. C. (1975) The problem-orientated record vs. the nursing care plan: a proposal. *Nursing Outlook,* **23** (8), 492-495

McKechnie A. M. & Miller N. R. (1971) The nursing care plan. *New Zealand Nursing Journal,* **64** (Dec.), 10-12

Malloy J. L. (1976) Taking exception to problem-oriented nursing care. *American Journal of Nursing,* **76** (4), 582-583

Marks-Maran D. J. (1979) Problem-orientated nursing care plans. *Medical Record,* **20** (2), May

Neal M. C. (1971) Workshops offer nurses opportunity to learn to write nursing care plans. *Hospital Topics,* **49** (Sept.), 29-31

Niland M. B. & Bentz P. M. (1974) A problem-oriented approach to planning nursing care. *Nursing Clinics of North America,* **6** (June), 235-245

Palisin H. E. (1971) Nursing care plans are a snare and a delusion. *American Journal of Nursing,* **71** (1), 63-66

Ryan B. J. (1973) Nursing care plans: a systems approach to developing criteria for planning and evaluation. *Journal of Nursing Administration,* **3** (May/June), 50-58

Stevens B. J. (1972) Why don't nurses write nursing care plans? *Journal of Nursing Administration,* **11** (Nov./Dec.), 6-7, 91

Wagner D. M. (1968) Care plans: right, reasonable and reachable. *American Journal of Nursing,* **68** (5), 986-990

Woody M. & Mallison M. (1973) The problem-oriented system for patient centred care. *American Journal of Nursing,* **73** (7), 1168-75

Zimmerman D. S. & Gohrke C. (1970) The goal-directed approach — it does work. *American Journal of Nursing,* **70** (2), 806-810

Primary nursing and total patient care

BOOKS

Johnston D. F. & Hood G. (1972) *Total Patient Care: Foundation and Practice.* St Louis: Mosby

Kraegel J. (1974) *Patient Care Systems.* Oxford: Blackwell Scientific Publications

Marram G. *et al.* (1974) *Primary Nursing: A Model for Individualized Care.* St Louis: Mosby

JOURNAL ARTICLES

Anderson M. (1976) Primary nursing in day-by-day practice. *American Journal of Nursing,* **76** (5), 802-805

Bakke K. (1974) Primary nursing: perceptions of a staff nurse. *American Journal of Nursing,* **74** (8), 1432-34

Brainerd S. & LaMonica E. L. (1975) A creative approach to individualized nursing. *Nursing Forum,* **14,** 188-193

Giske K. L. (1974) Primary nursing: an organisation that promotes professional practice. *Journal of Nursing Administration,* **4** (Jan./Feb.), 28-31

Giske K. L. (1974) Primary nursing: evaluation. *American Journal of Nursing,* **74** (8), 1436-38

Daeffler R. J. (1975) Patients' perceptions of care under team and primary care. *Journal of Nursing Administration,* **5** (Mar./Apr.) 20-26

Davies M. J. (1975) Total patient care assessments of student and pupil nurses during the community care option. *Nursing Mirror,* **140** (Feb. 6), 64-64

Fleming J. (1973) The secret of total patient care. *Nursing Mirror,* **136** (Jan. 5), 37

Isler C. (1976) Rx for a sick hospital: primary nursing care. *R. N. Magazine,* **39** (Feb.), 60-65, 67

Keane V. R. (1974) What are the challenges — the major elements of primary nursing care. *Hospital Topics,* **52** (Nov./Dec.), 43-46

Kocher P. (1976) Should primary nursing replace team nursing? *Nursing Care,* **9** (Feb.), 32-33

Logsdon A. (1973) Why primary nursing? *Nursing Clinics of North America,* **8** (June), 283-291

Manthey M. (1973) Primary nursing is alive and well in the hospital. *American Journal of Nursing,* **73** (1), 83-87

Manthey M. *et al.* (1970) Primary nursing. *Nursing Forum,* **9,** 65-83

Martin N. M. *et al.* (1973) Nurses who nurse. *American Journal of Nursing,* **73** (8), 1383-85

Matthews A. (1972) Total patient care in the wards. *Nursing Mirror,* **134** (Feb. 11), 29-31

Mundinger M. O. (1973) Primary nurse — rôle evaluation. *Nursing Outlook,* **21** (10), 642-645

Neuman B. M. & Young R. J. (1972) A model for teaching total patient approach to patient problems. *Nursing Research,* **21** (May/June), 264-269

Page M. (1974) Primary nursing — perceptions of a head nurse. *American Journal of Nursing,* **74** (8), 1435-36

Putt A. M. (1975) Letter commenting on: Patient perception of care under team and primary nursing, by R. J. Daeffler, J O

N A, Mar./April 1975. *Journal of Nursing Administration,* **5** (July/Aug.), 7, 11-12

Race G. A. (1974) T. P. C. A plan with R N's at the center. *R N Magazine,* **37** (April), 34-35

Rissler N. L. (1975) Development of an instrument to measure patient satisfaction with nurses and nursing care in primary care settings. *Nursing Research,* **24** (Jan./Feb.), 45-52

Robinson A. M. (1974) Primary care nursing at two teaching hospitals. *R N Magazine,* **47** (April), 31-34

Slater P. V. (1972) Nursing the whole patient. *Australian Nurses Journal,* **2** (Dec.), 25-29

Warrier P. (1972) Don't be ten years behind. *Nursing Mirror,* **134** (Feb. 4), 12

Patient-centred care

BOOKS

Abdellah F. G. *et al.* (1960) *Patient Centered Approaches to Nursing.* New York: Macmillan

Abdellah F. G. *et al.* (1973) *New Directions in Patient Centered Nursing.* New York: Macmillan

Matheney R. V. *et al.* (1972) *Fundamentals of Patient Nursing.* St Louis: Mosby

JOURNAL ARTICLES

Brinham R. O. J. (1975) Learning while caring. *Nursing Mirror,* **140** (May 22, 29), 81-82

Holloway A. J. (1974) Patient centred nursing care. *New Zealand Nursing Journal,* **68** (Sept.), 14-16

Hospitals (1973) Patient's rights — nursing responsibilities. *Hospitals,* **47** (June), 102-104

Kraegel J. M. (1972) A system of patient care based on patient needs. *Nursing Outlook,* **20** (4), 257-264

Lay J. (1972) Patient centred care. *Australian Nurses Journal,* **2** (Dec.), 30-32; *The Lamp,* (Dec.), 24-30

McDonnell C. (1972) What would you do? *American Journal of Nursing,* **72** (2), 296-301

McKay L. (1975) Do you practise what is taught? *New Zealand Nursing Journal,* **69** (July), 4-5

Richards A. C. (1975) Towards more patient centered care. *A O R N Journal,* **22** (Nov.), 782-785

Santorum C. D. & Sell V. M. (1973) A patient centered nursing service. *Journal of Nursing Administration,* **3** (July/Aug.), 32-40

Trent M. & Kramer M. (1972) The question behind the question. *Journal of Nursing Administration,* **2** (Jan./Feb.), 20-27

Patient allocation

JOURNAL ARTICLES

Bird K. (1974) Working with patient assignment. *Australian Nurses Journal,* **3** (May), 35-36

Correy M. F. (1976) Will patient assignment improve nursing care? *New Zealand Nursing Journal,* **69** (Feb.), 24-26

Jones E. S. (1977) A patient-allocation trial. *Nursing Times,* **73** (Mar. 17), 390-392

Jones W. L. (1977) Management by crisis or by objectives? Parts 1 & 2. *Nursing Times,* **73** (Mar. 10, 17), 342-343, 388-390

Kenny D. (1973) Patient assignment. *The Lamp,* **30** (Jan.), 17-18

Marks-Maran D. J. (1978) Patient allocation v. task allocation. *Nursing Times,* **74** (Mar. 25)

Matthews A. (1975) Patient allocation: a review. *Nursing Times,* **71** (July 10, 17, 24, 31), 65-79, occasional papers

Pembrey S. (1975) From work routines to patient assignment: an experiment in ward management. *Nursing Times,* **71** (Nov.), 1768-72

Team nursing

BOOKS

Douglass L. M. (1973) *Review of Team Nursing.* St Louis: Mosby

Newcomb D. P. & Swansburg R. C. (1971) *The Team Plan: A Manual for Nursing Service Administrators.* New York: Putnam

JOURNAL ARTICLES

Allen G. (1970) Team nursing's not new but it's satisfying. *New Zealand Nursing Journal,* **63** (Sept.), 5-9

Australian Nurses Journal (1971) The case of team nursing. *Australian Nurses Journal,* **1** (April), 38-40

Baumgart A. J. (1972) Are nurses ready for teamwork? *Canadian Nurse,* **68** (July), 19-20

Bergman R. (1974) Typology for teamwork. *American Journal of Nursing,* **74** (9), 1618-20

Etherington A. (1970) Team Nursing in the USA. *Nursing Times,* **66** (Jan. 22), 110-112

Forrest A. (1973) Modified team nursing. *Nursing Journal of India,* **44** (Aug.), 260, 263

Froebe D. (1974) Scheduling: by team or individually. *Journal of Nursing Administration,* **4** (May/June), 34-36

Germaine A. (1970) Problems of producing effective nursing teams. *Hospital Administration in Canada,* **12** (Mar.), 36, 38, 40

Germaine A. (1971) Applying the concept of team nursing. *Hospital Administration in Canada,* **13** (May), 58, 62-64

Germaine A. (1971) What makes team nursing tick. *Journal of Nursing Administration,* **1** (July/Aug.), 46-49

Germaine A. (1975) What method of nursing is best for you? *Hospital Administration in Canada,* **17** (Mar.), 34-36

Haren M. (1971) The practical experience of team nursing at St Vincent's Hospital. *The Lamp,* **28** (Oct.), 7, 9, 11, 13, 15

Kramer M. (1971) Team nursing — a means or an end? *Nursing Outlook,* **19** (10), 648-652

Kron T. (1971) Team nursing — how viable is it today? *Journal of Nursing Administration,* **1** (Nov./Dec.), 19-22

The Lamp (1973) Seminar on team nursing held at St Vincent's Hospital. *The Lamp,* **30** (Jan.), 7, 9, 11-16

Lawson O. (1975) Functional approach v. team nursing. *Nigerian Nurse,* **7** (July/Sept.), 10-14

Lio A. M. (1973) Leadership and responsibility in team nursing. *Nursing Clinics of North America,* **8** (June), 267-281

Marquand C. J. (1970) The core of team nursing. *New Zealand Nursing Journal,* **63** (Aug.), 9-10

Nelson M. C. (1972) Team nursing — what does it mean? *The Lamp,* **29** (Sept.), 15, 17, 19-20

Nolan M. (1974) Team nursing in the O R. *American Journal of Nursing,* **74** (2), 272-274

O'Brien R. A. (1975) Team nursing — an essential ingredient for success. *Australian Nurses Journal,* **5** (July), 39-40

Pembrey S. (1976) Teamwork in the ward. *Nursing Mirror,* **142** (April 8), 52-53

R N Magazine (1974) Speciality nursing teams in a small hospital. *R N Magazine,* **37** (Feb.), 34-35, 62, 63

Schultz L. & Yarmechuk M. (1972) 'Think in' at St Paul's Hospital. An annual workshop to revitalise team nursing. *Canadian Hospital,* **49** (March), 34-35

Sharp B. H. & Cross E. (1971) Rounds and rounds. *Nursing Outlook,* **19** (6), 419-420

Shepardson J. (1972) Team approach to the patient with cancer. *American Journal of Nursing,* **72** (3), 488-491

Stubber B. F. (1975) Team nursing — why? *Australian Nurses Journal,* **4** (April), 34-35; *Nursing Mirror,* **141** (Sept. 11), 72-73

Theis G. (1974) A change from team nursing. *Nursing Outlook,* **22** (April), 258-259

REPORT

Brogden G. H. (1974) *Project Report on Team Nursing.* Submitted to North-East Thames Regional Health Authority, Geriatric Nursing Liason Committee, 19 June. (Project carried out at St George's Hospital, Hornchurch.)

Care Plan Format (Psychogeriatric Ward)

Admission History
Problem List and Nursing Intervention
Progress Notes
Discharge Plan

WARD
Admission History

SOCIAL INFORMATION:
Name:
Address:
Age:
Religion:
Admission status:
Next of Kin:
Address — if different:

LIVING ACCOMMODATION: Live alone:
                        Share with others:
                        Local Authority flat/house:
                        Local Authority home:
                        Sheltered flat:
                        Other:

DEPENDENTS:
Do you have visitors?   Yes: No:
                           Who calls?
                           How often?

Community services: Meals on wheels:
                           Home help:
                           Day centres:
                           Luncheon clubs:
                           Others:

Financial support: Pension book:
                           Rent book:
                           TV rent book:
                           Other:

Who is taking care of   Relative:
    these?   Friend:
                           Hospital:

OTHER SIGNIFICANT OBSERVATIONS:

INFORMATION ABOUT ACTIVITIES FOR DAILY LIVING

DIET: Number of meals a day:
                             Special diet:
                             Food preferences:
                             Dislikes:
                             Fluid preferences:
                             Dislikes:

SLEEP: Normal sleep pattern:
                             Daytime naps:
                             If unable to sleep — what else helps?
                             Night sedation taken — if any:

URINARY: Frequency:
                             Incontinent:
                             Dysuria:
                             Nocturia:
                             Normal:

BOWEL MOVEMENTS: Daily:
                             Other:
                             Type of laxative:
                             How often?

MOBILITY: Unrestricted   limited
                             Walking:
                             Dressing:
                             Bathing :
                             Eating:

HEARING: Good:
                             Poor:
                             Wears aid:

VISION: Good:
                             Poor:
                             Wears glasses: always: for reading:

PHYSICAL: Health Problems:

ADDITIONAL SIGNIFICANT OBSERVATIONS:

INFORMATION ABOUT MENTAL HEALTH

GENERAL APPEARANCE: Very tidy:
                      Tidy:
                      Untidy:
                      Grubby:

HOBBIES/INTERESTS:

MOOD: Elated: Anxious:
                      Cheerful: Withdrawn:
                      Smiling: Agitated:
                      Distressed: Aggressive:
                      Miserable: Suspicious:
                      Irritable: Bland:
                      Sad: Apathetic:
                      Other:

THOUGHT CONTENT: Hallucinations:
                      Delusions:
                      Paranoid ideas:

ORIENTATION: Time:
                      Place:
                      Person:
                      Very Confused:
                      Slightly confused:
                      Slightly orientated:
                      Very orientated:

MOTOR ACTIVITY: Overactive:
                      Normal:
                      Lethargic:

SPEECH: Retarded:
                      Normal: Accelerated:

ATTITUDE TO BEING IN HOSPITAL:

ANY OTHER SIGNIFICANT OBSERVATIONS:

HISTORY OBTAINED FROM: TAKEN BY:
                                Date:
IF NOT PATIENT   Time:
— relationship to patient:

**PROBLEM LIST AND NURSING INTERVENTION
MRS AMY SMITH**

DATE DEFINED	NO	PROBLEMS	DATE RESOLVED
8.2.80	1	Difficulty in dressing and washing efficiently.	
8.2.80	2	Almost total absence of short-term memory.	
8.2.80	3	Disorientation in time and place, e.g: sometimes thinks she is in her old place of work and mistakes people around for those she once knew.	
8.2.80	4	Rapid mood swings: behaviour ranges between: a) Overactive, e.g: leaves the ward to 'go home'. and b) Apathetic and drowsy, e.g: at times can barely walk.	
18.2.80	5	Broken and infected areas on a) Right ankle. b) Neck. c) Blister on right heel. d) On lower parts of both legs.	
19.2.80	6	Dry mouth.	25.2.80
23.2.80	7	Fails to feed herself when in drowsy state.	
28.2.80	8	Poor fluid intake.	
28.2.80		Chest infection.	

DATE IMPLEMENTED	NO	INTERVENTION	DATE RESOLVED
8.2.80	1	Dressing programme, with encouragement to do as much as possible for herself.	
8.2.80	2	Constant reminders as to real situations.	
8.2.80	3	a) As with 2. b) Encourage to be 'sociable' by joining every group activity. c) 'Enjoys a guinness'.	
8.2.80	4	a) Constant observation 'as required' tranquillisers. b) Careful observation & assistance encouraging independence. a) & b) Ensure adequate diet and fluids: Chart.	
18.2.80	5	Daily saline baths. Areas covered with dry Telfa dressings.	b) Neck 23.2.80
19.2.80	6	a) To have at least one glass of fluid with meals. b) Oral hygiene as required, in particular before meals.	
23.2.80	7	Needs feeding and encouragement.	
28.2.80	8	a) Give 200 mls hourly by mouth. b) Mouth care, 4-hourly. c) Nurse per shift allocated to chat.	
28.2.80	9	a) Antibiotics, as prescribed. b) T P R twice daily. c) Suction as required.	

PROGRESS NOTES

DATE	NAME Mrs. Amy Sullivan	SIGNATURE
23.2.80		

AM   Got out of bed shivering. Is somewhat hypermanic —
      looking for the sergeant. Thinks she is at Poplar Police
      Station (where she used to work) and looking for the
      duster and brooms. Coat locked away to lessen tempta-
      tion for her to leave at the end of her day's work.

PM   Extraordinary change. Has been very helpful without
      being 'high'. Got on with the washing up in the kitchen
      very effeciently, came to fetch the key to lock up after-
      wards (exclaimed 'I though it was a police whistle') when
      I gave it to her.

NIGHT Sleeping at 2130 hours and has slept soundly through
      out the night.

24.2.80

AM   Sitting crossing and recrossing legs about every five sec-
      onds. It was noticed about 1530 hours that she was
      sweating — temp. 37·2 resp. 40, pulse 100. She was put
      to bed and seen by the duty doctor who prescribed
      Ampicillin. At 1800 hours, observations had dropped to
      normal.

DISCHARGE PLAN   Ward:

Target date for discharge:

Name of patient:

Home Address:

Next of Kin (+ address)

Place to which patient will be discharged:

1. Has patient been told of discharge plans?
   Does he/she understand the plans?
   What is his/her reaction to the plans?

2 Have the next of kin been informed of the patient's impending discharge?
   What part are they playing in the preparations?

   What part will they play in the life of the patient after discharge?

3 Have the following referrals been (a) made (b) confirmed. (Tick where relevant.)

   Community nurses   (a)   (b)   Home Help   (a)   (b)
   Day centre   (a)   (b)   Meals-on-wheels   (a)   (b)
   Day hospital   (a)   (b)   Laundry service   (a)   (b)

   Name and address of social worker:

   Has an application for Part III accommodation been made for the future?

4. Has an outpatient follow up appointment been made?
   Have TTA's been obtained?
   Has an EC10 form been completed?
   Has (a) Transport   (b) Escort home   been arranged?
   (Tick where appropriate.)
   Are his rent/pension book ready and on the ward for patient to take?

5. Comments:

Guide to Completing the Nursing History

Explanatory Leaflet for the Ward

The objective in using a Nursing Admission Sheet is to obtain all the necessary information about a patient in order to plan his nursing care. Some of the information will be obtained from the patient's medical notes, other information will come from the nurse's own observations of the patient, but the bulk of it will be obtained from the patient himself (or if this is impossible, from his relatives).

It is important that only a minimum of information should come from medical notes because the notes contain MEDICAL information and not NURSING information. For this reason they cannot be relied upon too heavily for information regarding nursing care. Some of the questions listed in this guide may seem self-explanatory but they are written to help learners understand the importance of asking questions properly and using the information received as a 'jumping off' point for other questions. After all, the more information that is recorded on the admission sheet, the more informed are the nurses looking after that patient and they are better able to pin-point his individual needs or problems. This is not to say that ward sisters have never received this sort of information from a patient. However, by having a Nursing Admission Sheet handy for all nurses to read and use, the learners (who, after all carry out a large proportion of the nursing care) are now given an opportunity to know a lot about the patients they are nursing.

This guide is written to correspond to the sections of the Nursing Admission Sheet.

Admission information

— There is, first of all, a place for the patient's sticky label to be attached. If the patient has no sticky labels in his notes or has come to the ward without notes, a space is provided in which the nurse can write the patient's name, record number, address, date of birth, and age. When a sticky label does arrive on the ward, it can be affixed to the sheet if desired.

— Date and time of admission can be recorded by the nurse when the patient arrives on the ward.

— The type of admission can be circled or in the case of a transfer, the place from where the patient was transferred can be recorded by the nurse when the patient arrives on the ward.

— The marital status of the patient and his religion can also be recorded, either from the medical notes or by asking the patient or his relatives.

Next of kin

— This information may be obtained from the patient's medical notes BUT it is

116

a good idea to verify the information from the patient or relatives to make sure it is accurate. Next of kin can change their address and telephone number, and the medical notes are often not up to date. If the patient's next of kin is not on the telephone, it is wise to find out if there is a close relative or friend who might be contacted by telephone should the need arise. Adequate space has been provided for a several telephone numbers should this be the case.

Speech difficulty/language barrier

— This can be filled in by the nurse, based upon her own observation of the patient. If the patient does not speak English, the admission information will have to be obtained from a relative or a friend. It is a good idea to find out from the relative or friend what language and dialect the patient does speak so that an interpreter can be called in should the need arise. Other speech difficulties which can be included are: (a) tracheostomy (b) cerebral vascular accident or (c) glossectomy.

Care at home

— Ask the patient the following questions:
— "Are you being seen or helped by a district nurse or social worker at home? If Yes, can you tell me her name?" It is then the nurse's responsibility to inform the ward social worker of this so she can inform the relevant people in the community nursing service or social services department of the patient's admission to hospital.
— "Do you receive any help from the social services such as meals on wheels or home help?" If Yes, the nurse should again inform the ward social worker so she can inform the relevant people. It is important to specify which particular type of social service is used; as this makes it considerably easier to plan the appropriate help on discharge. This also helps communication and co-operation between the nursing staff and hospital social workers.
— Ask the patient (or relative) what is the name of his GP. Do not get this information from the notes: it is included on the Nursing Admission Sheet as a double check to make sure that the name of the GP listed in the medical notes is actually the patient's present GP. Patients often change GP's and this information doesn't necessarily appear in the patient's medical notes.

Additional admission information

— A space is provided next to the patient's sticky label for the nurse to write in the name of the Consultant(s), the name of the House Officer and the patient's diagnosis. This is all information which can be obtained from the notes. However, it is important to remember that a diagnosis on a 'casualty card' may only be provisional — so be careful before writing in the diagnosis.

Operations on present admission/date performed

— This section is to be filled in when the specific operation(s) has been decided upon or performed. It should not be used for statements such as 'for operation on hip' or 'for appendicectomy'. The date of the operation should be included once the patient has had surgery.

Past medical history/operations

— This section causes some controversy amongst the ward sisters who participate in the use of the Nursing Admission Sheets. Some sisters agree that the nurses should get this information from the patient to provide a double check that all the information about the patient's past history is actually recorded. What has happened occasionally is that patients have forgotten to mention certain bits of information about their past medical history and the nurse has picked these ommissions up. Other ward sisters feel that the information is more accurate if it is just taken from the patient's medical notes and written in on the Admission Sheet. A compromise, perhaps, would be for the nursing staff to ask the patient if he has had any past illnesses or operations and write down what the patient says. The nurse can then go back to see if there is anything further in the notes that the patient has not told her. The nurse can then add these other bits of information, (if any) to what she has been told by the patient.

Allergies

— Medical staff, when taking their medical history from the patient, often ask him if he is allergic to any drugs. But, as nurses know well, patients can often be allergic to other things that come into the direct jurisdiction of nursing, such as plaster, certain foods, etc. The nurse, therefore, should ask: "Are you allergic to *anything*?"

History of present complaint

— The purpose of this section is to obtain a brief statement from the patient or his relatives about how long his present illness or problems have been troubling him. What was it that brought him to the doctor? Was it as the result of a long-standing complaint or an acute emergency? This should be a short comment so as to put his present complaint into perspective.

Other current health problems

— Patients can get the misguided idea that if they are in hospital for one problem, no one is really interested in any other health problems which they might have. If this happens, patients can undergo unnecessary suffering merely because they have a health problem other than that for which they have been admitted. The nurse should therefore, ask: "Do you have any other problems with your health other than (. . . reason for admission . . .)?"

What patient says is reason for admission

— This section is to find out whether there is a discrepancy between what the patient believes is the reason for his admission — and his diagnosis. If such a discrepancy exists, a decision can then be made on whether and how the patient should be made aware of his diagnosis.

Questions that might be helpful are:

"What has the doctor told you is the reason why you have come into hospital?"

"Has the doctor given you any idea of how long you will be in hospital?"

— Provision has been made here for the nursing staff to write down any regularly-occurring events or activities in the patient's day which they may want to be reminded about. These could include something like 'daily urine testing' but the section is really meant for things like 'goes to the gym every day at 2 p.m.' or 'No 999'. The nursing staff, however, can use this section for anything they find relevant.

Social history

— Ask the patient. "What is your occupation?" or "Do you have a job?"

— Ask, "Do you have any children?" If Yes, find out how old they are and if they still live at home. If the children are married with families of their own it may not be very relevant to include the information unless there is a problem, such as if they live too far away to visit often. This section on children is mainly for those patients who have young children and who may have a problem or worry about them as a result of their hospitalisation.

— Ask, "Do you have anyone else, such as elderly parents or relatives who you help to look after at home?"
BE SENSIBLE: if the patient has already told you that he is married, has two children at home but there is no problem about someone to look after them, and mum and dad live upstairs from the children, the question about whether or not the patient lives alone is irrelevant because he has already indirectly answered it. BUT if the patient has told you that he is single divorced or a widower, with no children or two children living in say, Edinburgh then the nurse should ask the patient if he lives alone.

— In addition to these questions one should ask for details about the patient's accommodation. This is important information to have in order to ensure that problems can be dealt with before a patient is discharged. Whether a patient has to walk up many flights of stairs, lives alone, or has no bathroom, are often critical factors in deciding when he can be discharged home. One should ask questions that are going to be relevant for that particular patient, eg. with an elderly patient who has had a hip replacement, the fact that he lives in a second-floor flat with no lift is important. So, one must naturally adapt the information required according to the patient's particular problems.

— Ask, "Are there any problems at home because you are in hospital such as paying rent or collecting pensions? "If Yes, the nurse must find out if the patient feels he would like to see a social worker to help him sort this out. Sister or Staff Nurse can then inform the social worker.

Visiting problems

— Ask, "Do your relatives/friends have any trouble visiting at the visiting times?" If Yes, "What is the trouble?" This information can then be passed on to Sister or Staff Nurse who can then make arrangements with the patient and his visitors about visiting outside the normal times.

Discharge planning

— The purpose of this section is twofold. Firstly, it enables all possible discharge arrangements to be made well before the patient is due to go home. Secondly, it allows improved communication among the nursing staff in knowing which discharge plans have been arranged and which still need to be sorted out.

— Once it is known approximately, if not definitely, when a patient will be ready to go home, the nursing staff can tick which type of discharge plans will be needed. If the patient has told you at the beginning of the admission interview that he was receiving a home help, or meals-on-wheels, then it is likely that he will need help from the social services when he goes home. So this part can be ticked on admission. Any other discharge needs should be ticked as well. When any one of the discharge plans has been organised, the date it was arranged should be inserted to let all concerned know what has been ordered or arranged — and what still needs to be done.

DAILY LIVING

This section elicits all the information about the patient's normal habits of daily living which enables the nurse to plan the care she will give that patient around what is normal for him. It also gives the nurse all the information which is solely related to NURSING aspects rather than medical aspects. This information enables the nurse to find out the individual needs of each patient.

Diet

— Ask: "Are you on any special diet?" If Yes, "What is it?" The nurse should also find out if the patient has been seen previously by the dietician.

— Ask: "Are there any foods which you don't like?" By finding this information out the nurse can make sure that the patient is not faced at mealtimes with a choice between only those things he dislikes.

— Ask: "Do you have a good or a poor appetite?" By finding this out, the nurse will know what size of portions to give that patient.

— Any remarks which the patient may make about his appetite or eating habits may also be recorded if they are relevant.

Sleep

— Ask: "How many hours do you usually sleep at night?" This question is necessary. How often does it happen that a patient wakes up at 4.00 a.m. and all the nursing staff think about is getting the doctor to prescribe night sedation to prevent it happening again? It may be that the patient wakes up at 4.00 a.m. because he has always woken at that time to go to work on the early shift.

— Ask: "Do you normally have to take any tablets to help you to sleep?" If Yes, find out what the tablets are. Should the patient need his sleeping tablets in hospital, the doctors can prescribe the tablets to which the patient is used.

Elimination

Bowels

— Ask: "Do you have any problems with your bowels?" If Yes, "What problems do you have?"
— Ask: "How often to you normally have your bowels open?"
— Ask: "Do you take any medication for your bowels?" This, again, is important so that if the patient needs medication for his bowels while he is in hospital, the doctors can, if possible, prescribe the same drug.

Urinary

— Ask: "Do you have any problems with passing water?" If the patient says that there are no problems, DON'T be content with just that bit of information. Continue by asking: "Do you have to get up in the night to pass water?" Very often the patient does not realise that this might be a problem or be abnormal. Any other comments the patient may make about his urinary output should also be recorded if they are relevant.

Female patients — menstruation

— The way these questions are asked depends upon the age of the patient. If the patient is young enough still to be having her menstrual periods, the following are suggestions of ways to ask the questions:
— "Are your monthly periods regular?"
— Do you have painful periods?" If Yes, find out what helps and write it under the remarks.
— "Do you take the Pill?"
— When is your next period due?" If the patient can't tell you when, you could ask: "When was your last period?"
— "Do you need us to get any ST's or tampons or can you supply them yourself?"
— Any remarks which the patient makes about her menstrual cycle should also be noted, if they are relevant. Also ask: "Do you have trouble with a vaginal discharge?"

  If the patient is elderly, the following are examples of questions you might ask:
— "You don't have your monthly periods anymore — can you tell me when they stopped coming?" This answer can be written in under remarks.
— "Have you had any bleeding or discharge since you have stopped having your monthly periods?" Any other remarks by the patient about them should also be recorded if they are relevant.

Hearing

— Ask: "How is your hearing?" If the patient says it is bad, find out if it is bad in both ears or only one ear — and which ear it is. If the patient's hearing is bad, find out if he has a hearing aid. If Yes, ask: "Do you have any problems with your hearing aid?"

Vision

— Ask: "How is your eyesight?" If the patient says that it is bad, find out whether one eye is bad or if both are. If the patient's eyesight is bad, find out if he wears glasses or contact lenses and whether it is at all times or only for reading.

Prosetheses/appliances/aids

— The questions in this section should only be asked if the patient has an obvious prosethesis or appliance or aid, and are NOT to be asked of all patients. But if the patient does have an artificial leg, breast prostheses, surgical corset, walking frame, tripod, etc., write down the type of appliance and ask: "Do you need any help with your (. . . type of appliance . . .)?"

Mobility

— This section is also one which may not need to be filled in. It will depend on the patient. If a patient is admitted to your ward, walks in unaided, is up and about, bathes himself etc. there is NO need to ask any of the questions in this MOBILITY section. Simply circle or tick No.

— If, however, the patient comes in on a trolley, or a wheelchair, or has a walking stick or walking frame, or it is obvious that he has a mobility problem, ask the questions in the following way:

— "I see you have problems with (. . . eg. walking/getting out of bed . . .). Do you have any trouble doing anything else, such as: (. . . dressing, feeding . . . etc.)?"

— In this way, all nurses become aware of exactly what help the patient needs. If we know this, other health care professionals such as the occupational or physiotherapists can be called in to help the patient with the things he cannot do on his own.

— Do more that just tick the relevant word or words which are listed in this section — it is better to include as concise a description as you possibly can of the exact mobility needs of the patient.

Oral

— Ask: "Do you have any problems with your mouth or teeth?" If Yes, "Can you tell me about it?"

— Ask: "Do you wear dentures?" If Yes, "Are they top and bottom dentures? Do you have any problems with your dentures?"

— Ask: "Are any of your teeth crowned?"

— The nurse should also use her own observations of the patient's mouth as it appears to her during the course of the interview and record any problems she may observe.

NURSES OBSERVATIONS

This is a fairly open-ended section and is completed partly by asking a question of the patient and partly by observing 'non-verbal' signs which the patient may be showing that tell you how he really feels. The nurse may circle any of the three words listed if they describe her opinion of the patient's attitude. The rest of the section has been left blank for you to assess the patient's own reaction to being in hospital and any social, cultural or environmental factors which could contribute to his attitude. In this way the nurse understands why the patient may be reacting the way he is and can see the patient in terms of being a person and not just a name and a diagnosis and a bed number.

— Ask: "How do you feel about being in hospital?" Write down the patient's answer but also take note of anything in his manner or behaviour which may tell you something more, or something different from what he has said. The nurse can also include whether or not she feels that the patient's attitude is caused by his admission or by other things.

— The nurse might also ask how the patient sees himself. Is he normally mentally and physically active? And if so, does the absence of mental of physical activity while in hospital worry him. The nurse should find out if the patient sees himself as a 'loner' or as someone who likes having people round him all the time. She should try to ascertain whether or not the patient feels helpless in hospital or otherwise distressed or worried. Does the patient seem to know what is his expected behaviour and what he should or should not do in hospital? How these questions are phrased really depends upon the type of patient and the situation.

— Remember: The nurse must avoid putting down her own thoughts or biases and concentrate on what the patient is saying and what behaviour is being shown.

THIS IS THE LAST ACTUAL QUESTION TO BE ASKED OF THE PATIENT. THE REMAINDER OF THE SHEET SHOULD BE COMPLETED AWAY FROM THE BEDSIDE.

General appearance

— Circle any of the words which describe, in your opinion, what the patient's appearance seems to be. If you circle something other than 'normal' — please describe in the space provided his appearance as indicated by any other word you have circled. Be as specific and descriptive as possible.

Skin

— Circle any of the words which describe to you the appearance of the patient's skin. If you find out more about the condition of the patient's skin in the next few days through baths and pressure area care, please come back and add any information to this section. Again, if word other than 'satisfactory' is circled, please write in any further descriptions and be as specific as possible.

Level of consciousness

— Circle the word which describes the patient's state of consciousness on admission. If word other than 'orientated' is circled, write in any further information in the space provided.

Information received from and by

Write in who has given you all the information (ie. patient, patient's wife, etc.).
Sign your own name and, where applicable, include your level of seniority such as
your set number or the year you are in.

— Write the date and time that the information was obtained.

POINTS TO REMEMBER

It is not necessary to take an admission interview as soon as the patient has been
admitted. In many cases it is better to wait a day or two until the patient has had a
chance to settle into the ward before obtaining this information. Do not bother to
take the information if you are not going to use it! Also, please remember to write
'no' or 'not applicable' in a section rather than leave it blank. This provides a
means of ensuring that the questions within that section were asked.

If the patient is unable to give you the information because he speaks no
English, or is not well enough, this is NO EXCUSE for not getting the information.
Relatives must be asked in the patient's stead. Of course, there will be circums-
tances where no relatives are available, but most of the time there is a relative
who can be approached for the information.

So far, no patient has refused to be interviewed for the purpose of getting this
information, but if ever it should happen that a patient does not want to supply
this information, do not try to force him. Just leave him be and let Sister or Staff
Nurse know the situation.

Appendix 3

Leaflet for Ward Staff Introducing Nursing Care Plans as part of Nursing Research Project

Introduction

The nursing research project is an experimental use of Nursing Care Plans based on *the nursing process*. The nursing process is a topic that is very much in the news at the moment, and much discussion is taking place about whether it can be implemented and care plans written as part of the normal ward routine.

What is care planning?

Care planning uses a problem-solving approach. The nursing process provides the theoretical framework within which care planning is developed. This approach enables nurses to develop a more questioning attitude to nursing care so that nursing practices and procedures are not continued 'because they have always been done this way' but because they have been proved to be effective.

What has happened so far?

The first stage of the project was the introduction and use of the *Nursing Admission Sheet* as a means of assessing patient's needs in more detail and more systematically. Such an assessment is essential if the nurse is to have sufficient information with which to identify the patient's nursing problems and plan his care. The next stage was the introduction and use of a new-style *Progress Record* to replace the old Kardex, and finally, we have started on the third stage, namely the writing of *Care Plans*.

The Nursing Care Plans

Each Nursing Care Plan has three components: Nursing Admission Sheet; Progress Record; and Care Plan. The Care Plan for each patient is kept in a ring folder so that all the information about a patient is in one place.

The *Nursing Admission Sheet* is in use in 8 wards so it may already be familiar to you. If it is unfamiliar you should read the *Guide to Completing the Nursing Admission Sheet,* a copy of which is kept on the ward. The Research Team will also give talks about how to complete the form to those who have not had a teaching session either while in School or while on another ward. It is very important that you know what to do, so ask for help or for teaching if you need them.

The *Progress Record* is the equivalent of the Kardex on the other wards, although it is filled in differently. It has TWO sections, the first for recording what has happened to the patient, and the second for any special instructions about what is to happen to the patient. NO instructions should be written in the progress section. You will be expected to write the reports on your own patients, which may be something that you are not used to doing on other wards. If you don't know what to write then ask Sister or Staff Nurse for advice and they will help you.

The *Care Plan* is a problem-orientated plan of care tailored to meet the needs of a particular patient. On it are listed the patient's nursing problems, the goal for each problem and the nursing instructions to meet that goal. You will be expected to write nursing care plans but ONLY after you have been shown how to do so either by Sister, Staff Nurse or the Research Team. The Plan will always be checked by the nurse in charge (usually Sister) to see that it contains all the necessary instructions. Many of the Plans will in fact be written by Sister or Staff Nurse, and you will have to read them and carry out the care that they have ordered.

Why write Care Plans?

A Care Plan provides you with all the information you need to give the nursing care which the trained staff have decided is the best care for that patient. The Plan is detailed and explicit so that everyone knows exactly what should be done and how it should be done. The emphasis is on the contribution that nursing can make to the patient's comfort and progress.

These Care Plans are experimental. Their use will be continued for a period and we will then review the situation. So that we can assess their usefulness accurately it is important they they are given a proper trial, so a Plan should be written for every patient.

Care Plans and patient allocation

Care planning emphasises the needs of each patient as an individual. It works best, therefore, when one nurse cares for the same group of patients providing total care for them, ie. PATIENT ALLOCATION. Research has shown that patients and nurse find patient allocation more satisfying. Sister tries to allocate the same group of patients to you for several days at a time so that you really have a chance to get to know them properly. Obviously, if there are patients who are particularly difficult to nurse you will not be left to struggle on trying to cope with them — everyone will share the load. The nurse to whom a patient is allocated is, therefore, responsible for the total care of that patient. This means that you will not only carry out the care as ordered on the Care Plan, but also update the Plan when appropriate, write the progress notes and hand over to the nurse looking after the patient during the next shift. This may seem a lot of responsibility but if you are unsure about any of it you can, and should ask for help. Every effort will be made to see that you are taught how to do things, and in fact the nurses so far have not found any great difficulty in doing them.

What are the advantages of the new system?

The nursing process has already been included in the nurse training syllabus by the General Nursing Council, and questions are being asked which emphasise this approach. You will be among the few who have actually used the nursing process. Both the third and fourth assessments are based on the idea of planning care, so your experience in this ward should help you with those. Care studies and essays now emphasise care planning and planning care to meet the individual needs of each patient. Again, your experience with the Nursing Care Plans will be very useful

In the longer term the use of Nursing Care Plans will help us to build up knowledge about nursing and about the effect that nursing has upon the patients. Such knowledge will be of immense value to nursing in general and to nursing research, and will enable nurses to identify the most effective care for specific nursing problems or particular groups of patients.

Summary

We hope that you will enjoy participating in the project and using the Nursing Care Plans. Their success or failure is in your hands. We find them very exciting and hope that you will at least find them useful in your work on the wards and in the School. We want to know what you think of them; we will be asking you for suggestions and criticisms — and praise — so if you want them altered it is up to you.

Essential reading

1   The Guide to the Nursing Admission Sheet.
2   The leaflet explaining the Nursing Research Project.
3   Rediscovering the patient. *Nursing Times,* Nov. 30 1978
4   Rheumatology — a team approach. *Nursing Mirror,* Nov. 30 1978
5   The nursing process. *Nursing Times,* June 1977
Copies of all these leaflets and articles are available on the ward

Learning objectives

Just as objectives are important in care planning, so they are also in relation to your own learning.
Suggested objectives for care planning are:

(i)   you should be able to explain what is meant by (a) care planning (b) the nursing process.
(ii)   you should be able to complete a Nursing Admission Sheet.
(iii)   you should be able to identify the patients' nursing problems.
(iv)   you should be able (with help) to write a Nursing Care Plan.
(v)   you should be able to write the daily progress report on your own patients, as well as being able to give a verbal report on them.

Jennifer Hunt
SNO (Research)

Index